The Cholesterol Controversy

The Cholesterol Controversy

Gilbert Thompson

Emeritus Professor of Clinical Lipidology,
Department of Metabolic Medicine,
Imperial College, Hammersmith Hospital, London

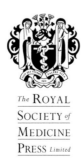

The ROYAL
SOCIETY *of*
MEDICINE
PRESS *Limited*

© 2008 Royal Society of Medicine Press Ltd

Published by the Royal Society of Medicine Press Ltd
1 Wimpole Street, London W1G 0AE, UK
Tel: +44 (0)20 7290 2921
Fax: +44 (0)20 7290 2929
Email: publishing@rsm.ac.uk
Website: www.rsmpress.co.uk

British Library Cataloguing in Publication Data
A catalogue record for this book is available from the British Library

ISBN 978-1-85315-802-5

Distribution in Europe and Rest of World:	Distribution in the USA and Canada:
Marston Book Services Ltd	Royal Society of Medicine Press Ltd
PO Box 269	c/o BookMasters Inc
Abingdon	30 Amberwood Parkway
Oxon OX14 4YN, UK	Ashland, OH 44805, USA
Tel: +44 (0)1235 465500	Tel: +1 800 247 6553/+1 800 266 5564
Fax: +44 (0)1235 465555	Fax: +1 419 281 6883
Email: direct.order@marston.co.uk	Email: order@bookmasters.com

Distribution in Australia and New Zealand:

Elsevier Australia
30-52 Smidmore Street
Marrickville NSW 2204, Australia
Tel: +61 2 9517 8999
Fax: +61 2 9517 2249
Email: service@elsevier.com.au

Typeset by Saxon Graphics Ltd
Printed in the UK by Bell & Bain, Glasgow

Contents

Foreword

Professor Gilbert Thompson has had a wide-ranging career in clinical science. Following his medical studies at St Thomas's Hospital, he served for 5 years in the Royal Army Medical Corps. While posted to Ghana, and with encouragement from Herman Lehmann, he made his own electrophoresis apparatus and carried out studies of the haemoglobinopathies of West Africa, work which formed the basis of his thesis for the MD of London University. With this background, it was not surprising that, in 1963, when he left the Army, he had no difficulty in obtaining a post at Hammersmith Hospital, then a leading centre for clinical research. There he encountered a patient with severe osteomalacia due to intestinal malabsorption, and this led to his development, with Barry Lewis, of tritium-labelled vitamin D for studies of absorption. Their work was published in the prestigious *Journal of Clinical Investigation*.

By then, clinical investigators were beginning to realize that lipids, and particularly cholesterol, were involved in the development of coronary heart disease. It was at that time that butter and cream came to be banned from the dining tables of believers and the craze for jogging began. Gilbert Thompson, already influenced by his work at Hammersmith, was further stimulated to an interest in plasma lipids by meeting the future Nobel laureates, M. Brown and J. Goldstein, during a year's secondment to the Massachusetts General Hospital. He went on to devote himself to working full-time on lipids and their relationship to coronary heart disease.

He had the good fortune to be supported by the Medical Research Council. Nevertheless, there were many contemporary cardiologists on both sides of the Atlantic who vehemently rejected the idea that cholesterol had anything to do with the lipid deposits that accumulated in the blood vessels and thus caused coronary artery disease. In the USA, there was considerable controversy, and in Britain during the 1970s the attack on the cholesterol hypothesis was led by some of the most distinguished cardiologists in the land. They included Sir John McMichael, legendary head of the Department of Medicine at Hammersmith until his retirement in 1966.

Gilbert Thompson is a man of great determination who has been neither afraid of controversy nor able to resist a challenge – after all, he ran in both the London and New York marathons while in his sixties. In this book, he describes how he enthusiastically entered the fray. It was the King in *Alice in Wonderland*, who advised: "Begin at the beginning.... And go on till you come to the end; then stop". Thompson has done just that. He describes how he played a role in scientific debates and used his nimble pen to support his own side of the argument. With the development of the statins, which so remarkably control levels of cholesterol in the blood and which also reduce cardiac mortality, he feels entirely vindicated in his views. It is sad that his main opponents, already in retirement at the time when the controversy was at its height, did not live to witness what he regards as the final denouement. The discovery of statins merits, in his view, a Nobel Prize just as much as any of the great scientific achievements of our age.

Christopher Booth

Preface

The growth of knowledge depends entirely on disagreement.

This quotation from Karl Popper features on the website of the International Network of Cholesterol Skeptics, a group of individuals who refute the concept that cholesterol plays a causal role in atherosclerosis and reject the evidence that lowering blood cholesterol with diet or drugs reduces the risk of cardiovascular disease. They represent the dying embers of a controversy which started in the 1950s, reached its peak in the 1970s and 1980s, and then subsided in the 1990s, the controversy seemingly being resolved by the positive outcome of the Scandinavian Simvastatin Survival Study, or 4S. This was the first in a series of prevention trials using statins which showed that lowering cholesterol reduced both cardiovascular events and total mortality. During the preceding years, there had been a great deal of disagreement among those involved in research into atherosclerosis, but the concomitant growth in knowledge was even greater, eventually resulting in what could be described as a favourable light-to-heat ratio. Consequently, there is no longer any doubt that lowering cholesterol reduces the risk of heart attacks and strokes – the only question that remains is by how much it needs to be lowered to achieve the optimal benefit.

The cholesterol controversy raged just as fiercely on the other side of the Atlantic and is described in *The Cholesterol Wars* by Dan Steinberg, Professor of Medicine at the University of California San Diego and the doyen of lipid research in the USA. The present account focuses primarily on the events and people involved in the controversy in Britain, many of whom are still alive and whose straight-from-the-horse's-mouth comments were published recently in the form of a Wellcome Witness Seminar entitled 'Cholesterol, Atherosclerosis and Coronary Disease in the UK, 1950–2000'. The meeting was organized and chaired by Professor Michael Oliver, who has actively participated on both sides of the cholesterol debate from its inception to its conclusion. The transcripts of that meeting provide a valuable source of information, much of it never previously published. However, several of the most severe critics of the lipid hypothesis, such as Sir John McMichael and Professor Tony Mitchell, are now deceased, and one must therefore rely upon published documents and personal recollections to reflect the views they held during their lifetime.

This book is aimed mainly at physicians and other health-care workers interested in the treatment and prevention of cardiovascular disease, including those in the pharmaceutical industry. Here and there, its narrative overlaps with that of my earlier book *Hammersmith Marathon*, but only to a very limited extent. The controversy over the lipid hypothesis (the concept that cholesterol circulating in the blood gets sequestered within the arterial wall to form atheromatous plaques that cause coronary heart disease) involved cardiologists, epidemiologists, lipidologists, pathologists and nutritionists, and its history is particularly relevant to those who are working or have worked in these fields. However, cholesterol has had such a high public profile in recent years that the book might also interest scientifically knowledgeable laypersons, especially those taking one of the statin drugs or a functional food to lower their cholesterol. In terms of importance, the discovery of the statins has been likened to that of penicillin, but, unlike Alexander Fleming, the Nobel Prize has still to be awarded to Akira Endo, the man who discovered the first statin.

Having started with a quotation, it seems appropriate to conclude the Preface with another, this one from Maynard Keynes: 'There is no harm in being sometimes wrong – especially if one is promptly found out.' Unfortunately for the many patients who had high cholesterol levels and heart disease at the time, it took the best part of 50 years to disprove the sceptics and demonstrate that lowering cholesterol both reduced risk and was safe. This book relates why it took so long.

List of illustrations

Acknowledgements

I am indebted to the following friends and colleagues for providing me with information about past events and for their helpful comments on parts of the manuscript: Professor John Betteridge, Sir Christopher Booth, Professor John Hampton, Professor Malcolm Law, Dr Nicolas Myant, Dr Rossi Naoumova, Professor Michael Oliver, Professor Tom Sanders, Dr Michael Schachter, Dr Mary Seed and Professor James Shepherd. I also wish to thank Caroline Davidson for her constructive literary criticisms, Liz Manson for her help with the technical aspects of the manuscript and Hannah Wessely for her skilful editing.

I am especially grateful to Sir Christopher Booth for agreeing to write the Foreword. He does so from a unique perspective, having been my first mentor at the Hammersmith and later the successor to Sir John McMichael as Director of the Department of Medicine. He is also a distinguished historian and was Harveian Librarian at the Royal College of Physicians between 1989 and 1997. His rather guarded acceptance of the lipid hypothesis probably reflects his belief that the unexpected can always occur in science and trip one up. In other words, it may be that as far he is concerned the Fat Lady has not yet sung.

Last but certainly not least, this book would never have seen the light of day had it not been for donations from McNeil Nutritionals Ltd and Raisio Nutrition Ltd, Finland, which helped defray the costs of publication. Their generosity is greatly appreciated.

CHAPTER 1

The beginnings of the controversy

Cardiologists reject early data on coronary risk factors

Chapter summary

- Lipids irrelevant to cardiology

- Role of epidemiology rejected

- An uncompromising environment for research

I t is hard to pin down the precise origin of the cholesterol controversy in Britain, but a tenuous case can be made for its being conceived in the competitive environment of the Postgraduate Medical School at Hammersmith Hospital (Figure 1.1) after the Second World War. The Department of Medicine there was dominated by cardiologists, the most notable being John McMichael, the Professor of Medicine, and his first assistants, Paul Wood and Peter Sharpey-Schafer. There was a rather left-wing atmosphere about the place and free speech flourished. Legendary altercations reputedly took place between Sharpey-Schafer, educated at Winchester, King's College, Cambridge, and University College Hospital, London, and Wood, who had trained in Melbourne and had an Antipodean lack of respect for the Establishment.[1] Like his famous grandfather, Sir Edward Sharpey-Shafer FRS, Peter Sharpey-Shafer was intolerant of those he considered intellectually inferior[2] whereas Wood was scornful of his colleague's lack of clinical experience in cardiology.

Sharpey-Shafer left the Hammersmith scene in 1948 when he was appointed Professor of Medicine at St Thomas's Hospital. As a medical student there in the early 1950s, I remember attending a ward round he conducted in complete silence, his only interest seemingly being to inspect his patients' necks to ascertain which of them had a raised jugular venous pressure, and also an evening when he had been invited to a party held in a fellow medical student's flat. On arrival, he said, 'Sorry I'm late – my wife's just aborted', and sank into an armchair behind a newspaper. He seemed oblivious to what was going on around him until someone spotted the lens of a camera poking through a

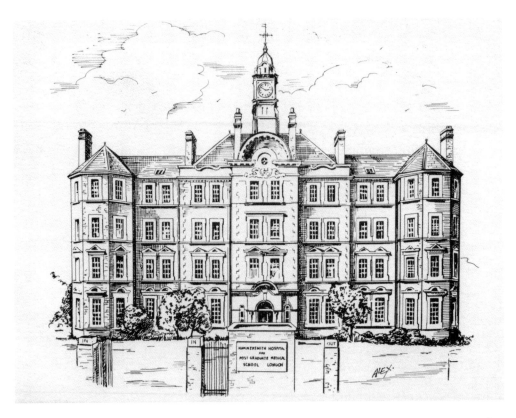

Figure
1.1 *Hammersmith Hospital and Postgraduate Medical School in the 1960s (from a Christmas card sold by the Friends of Hammersmith Hospital)*

hole in the newspaper, recording our antics to show to his friends! His death in 1963, aged only 55, was described by McMichael as a unique loss.[2]

Paul Wood left the Hammersmith a year after Sharpey-Shafer, in 1949, when he was invited to set up the Institute of Cardiology at the National Heart Hospital and teach clinical cardiology to postgraduates. His book *Diseases of the Heart and Circulation*, published in 1950, was a 'must' in those days for anyone aspiring to pass the examination for membership of the Royal College of Physicians. According to Michael Oliver,[3] the first edition contains the earliest British reference to the relationship between cholesterol and coronary heart disease, namely that 'considerations should be given to the possibility that raised cholesterol might result from coronary heart disease'. This comment probably reflected Wood's preoccupation with the manifestations of cardiac disease rather than its causes.

Lipids irrelevant to cardiology

In 1953, Michael Oliver, then a young cardiologist at the Edinburgh Royal Infirmary, and George Boyd, a biochemist at

Edinburgh University, reported the findings of a study of 200 patients with coronary disease and an equal number of control subjects at a meeting of the British Cardiac Society in Newcastle. Their results showed that plasma cholesterol levels were significantly higher in the coronary patients, the first time this had been demonstrated in the UK. However, there was total silence after Oliver's presentation, and not a question was asked during the discussion period. The silence was broken eventually by Paul Wood, who commented that this was irrelevant to cardiology.[4] That remark reflected the abrasively intolerant side of Wood's character, although he had many compensatory virtues,[1] while the absence of questions from the audience was indicative of the complete lack of interest in lipids among British cardiologists at that time. In the years ahead, however, apathy would be replaced by heated debate.

Undeterred, Oliver and Boyd pursued their research into lipids, using paper electrophoresis to separate the different classes of lipoproteins present in serum. They showed that patients with coronary disease not only had higher levels of total cholesterol than controls[5] but also that the distribution of lipoprotein classes was abnormal, with an excess of β-lipoprotein and a dearth of α-lipoprotein.[6] In today's jargon, their patients had a high ratio of low-density lipoprotein (LDL) to high-density lipoprotein (HDL) cholesterol, now a well accepted risk factor for coronary disease but a novel finding in those days. However, their next research venture was less successful, involving the administration of estrogens to men with coronary disease. Although this treatment lowered serum cholesterol, it had feminizing side-effects and failed to reduce coronary events.[7]

Paul Wood and George Boyd both died from coronary disease before they reached 60, an all too common event in those days. Wood had explicitly stated that he was not to be resuscitated, and therefore no attempt to do so was made when his heart arrested. The photograph of him in the published account of the first Paul Wood Lecture, established in his honour by the British Cardiac Society, shows a lean, quizzical-looking man holding a telltale cigarette between his fingers.[1] His death in 1962 at the age of 55 shocked cardiologists across the country, but, as he himself had said, he enjoyed living dangerously. He took risks and unfortunately paid the price.

The antipathy towards lipids felt by many cardiologists in those days was not entirely of their own making. This point is illustrated by a review article published in 1960, which, although it provided a cautious and balanced account of what was known at that time about the role of cholesterol in atherosclerosis, contained an unfortunate *embarras de richesses* of technical information.[8] It is unlikely that many cardiologists would have read any further than the third paragraph, which stated:

> The plasma lipids currently estimated in investigations into atherosclerosis are triglycerides and chylomicra, total (esterified and unesterified) cholesterol, phospholipids, alpha- and beta-lipoproteins and their sub-divisions and, more recently, the fatty acid composition of plasma and of ester cholesterol.

Edinburgh was not the only centre where lipid-related research in Britain was undertaken during the 1950s, another being Oxford. Brian Bronte-Stewart, a Cape Town graduate, was one of several immigrants from South Africa who made contributions to atherosclerosis research in Britain. When he first arrived, he worked with George Pickering at St Mary's Hospital in London, but he moved to Oxford when Pickering was appointed Regius Professor in 1956. Bronte-Stewart had started his research in Cape Town, where he, John Brock (Professor of Medicine in Cape Town) and Ancel Keys (the American epidemiologist) demonstrated differences in serum cholesterol between racial groups, which they attributed to differences in animal fat intake. Bronte-Stewart went on to show that differing death rates from coronary heart disease in various European countries, including Britain, correlated better with the hard:liquid fat ratio of the diet than with the total fat intake.[9] He also showed that when vegetable oils are hydrogenated they lose their cholesterol-lowering ability. In 1961, he was appointed Director of the newly established Medical Research Council (MRC) Atheroma Research Unit in Glasgow, but he tragically died from cancer 4 years later, aged only 42.

Another research worker in Oxford was Hugh Sinclair, an engagingly eccentric Fellow of Magdalen College, who was Reader in Human Nutrition and directed the Laboratory of Human Nutrition there for many years. In 1972, he established the International Institute of Human Nutrition on his estate at Sutton Courtenay, Abingdon. He, too, was interested in the role of diet in atherosclerosis but did not subscribe to the traditional view that a high-fat diet caused high serum cholesterol, which in turn caused atherosclerosis, which in turn caused coronary disease. His opposition was based to a large extent on his knowledge of Eskimos, whose fat intake was extremely high but in whom coronary disease was uncommon. Since most of their fat is polyunsaturated, Sinclair proposed that it was the relative deficiency of essential (polyunsaturated) fatty acids in Western diets that was atherogenic, rather than the high intake of total fat.[10] He went on to postulate that a high ratio of non-essential to essential fatty acids in the diet promoted fatty streaks in the arterial wall by increasing the proportion of cholesterol ester-ified with oleic acid (a non-essential fatty acid with one double bond) at the expense of linoleic acid (an essential fatty acid with two double bonds).[11] He summarized this concept in mock Shakespearean verse:

Oh, infarcted English,
Whose blood is full of saturated fats,
Cholesterol whose esters with wrong lipids
Have in these parts accumulated thus
Insoluble for lack of double bonds.

(Personal communication)

Sinclair's interest in the effects of the Eskimo diet was such that he lived for 3 months on food derived entirely from marine sources, consisting mainly of seal meat. He then analysed the resulting changes in the fatty acid composition of his plasma lipids, platelets and various tissues obtained by biopsy, including a testicular biopsy,[12] but his bleeding time was so prolonged that the liver biopsy he requested was ruled out as too dangerous. Although Sinclair's theory that atherosclerosis is a form of essential fatty acid deficiency was not substantiated by the evidence, his belief in the benefits of ω-3 fatty acids and the harmful effects of trans-fatty acids resulting from hydrogenation of oils is now increasingly accepted.

Role of epidemiology rejected

Apart from lipidology, another discipline which got short shrift from the Hammersmith cardiologists was epidemiology. The two may in fact have been unpopular for the same reason, in that both involved measurements performed in large groups or populations rather than individuals. This was the dawn of cardiac catheterization, and McMichael and his colleagues boldly exploited the technique to advance knowledge of cardio-vascular haemodynamics by detailed studies in small numbers of subjects. To their minds, that was how real clinical research should be conducted.

In 1953, Jerry Morris, then Director of the MRC Social Medicine Unit and regarded by many as the founding father of cardiovascular epidemiology in Britain, came up with some novel findings which suggested a link between coronary disease and exercise at work. He and his colleagues discovered that fatal heart attacks occurred less frequently in London bus conductors than in drivers and less often in postmen than in sedentary civil servants, findings which created a considerable stir when they were published.[13,14] Before they came out, however, he was advised by the Secretary of the MRC, Sir Harold Himsworth, to show the data to John McMichael. He did so and went on to suggest to the latter that epidemiology could play a useful role in supplementing clinical observation and laboratory experiments. According to Morris, McMichael listened carefully until he had finished and then retorted 'Rubbish!'[15] In sharp contrast, the Director of the US National Heart and Lung Institute flew over from Bethesda, Maryland, to discuss the possibility of a follow-up study, and Paul Dudley White, the doyen of American cardiologists, phoned from Boston to congratulate him. Morris stated that McMichael 'came round in later years',[15] but there was no sign of this after 20 years, when he again rejected the concept that exercise had a protective effect and criticized 'the unfortunate separation of epidemiology from close clinical analysis of the data',[16] the implication being that only the latter could reveal causal relationships.

An uncompromising environment for research

This, then, was the uncompromising environment confronting those interested in carrying out research into coronary disease in Britain at the start of the 1960s. Although the statistics showed that this disorder was the commonest cause of death in both men and women, little was being done in the way of prevention apart from discouraging smoking. The only other risk factor taken seriously was blood pressure, hypertension being a topic of particular interest to McMichael at the Hammersmith and Pickering at Oxford. The 1950s and 1960s were the heyday of clinicians in the National Health Service, who effectively ran it, and at the top of the tree were academic cardiologists such as McMichael and Pickering. Lipids were generally considered to be of minor importance and regarded as the concern of laboratory-based biochemists, not of practising physicians. However, although the future for those interested in the role of lipids in atherosclerosis looked decidedly unpromising at that stage, the situation gradually improved with the passage of time – but only after much controversy.

References

1. Somerville J. The master's legacy: the first Paul Wood lecture. *Heart* 1998; **80**: 612–19.
2. Obituary: Edward Peter Sharpey-Shafer. *Br Heart J* 1964; **26**: 430–2.
3. Cholesterol, atherosclerosis and coronary disease in the UK, 1950–2000. In Reynolds LA, Tansey EM, eds. *Wellcome Witnesses to Twentieth Century Medicine* 2006; **27**: 4.
4. Cholesterol, atherosclerosis and coronary disease in the UK, 1950–2000. In Reynolds LA, Tansey EM, eds. *Wellcome Witnesses to Twentieth Century Medicine* 2006; **27**: 7.
5. Oliver MF, Boyd GS. The plasma lipids in coronary artery disease. *Br Heart J* 1953; **15**: 387–92.
6. Oliver MF, Boyd GS. Serum lipoprotein patterns in coronary sclerosis and associated conditions. *Br Heart J* 1955; **17**: 299–302.
7. Oliver MF, Boyd GS. Influence of reduction of serum lipids on prognosis of coronary artery diseases – a five-year study using oestrogen. *Lancet* 1961; **2**: 499–505.
8. Oliver MF. Plasma lipids and atherosclerosis. *Proc R Soc Med* 1960; **53**: 15–18.
9. Bronte-Stewart B. The effect of dietary fats on the blood lipids and their relation to ischaemic heart disease. *Br Med Bull* 1958; **14**: 243–52.
10. Sinclair HM. Deficiency of essential fatty acids and atherosclerosis, etcetera. *Lancet* 1956; **270**: 381–3.
11. Sinclair HM. Prevention of coronary heart disease: the role of essential fatty acids. *Postgrad Med J* 1980; **56**: 579–84.
12. Sinclair HM. The relative importance of essential fatty acids of the linoleic and linolenic families: studies with an Eskimo diet. *Prog Lipid Res* 1981; **20**: 897–9.
13. Morris JN, Heady JA, Raffle PA, et al. Coronary heart-disease and physical activity of work. *Lancet* 1953; **265**: 1053–7.
14. Morris JN, Heady JA, Raffle PA, et al. Coronary heart-disease and physical activity of work. *Lancet* 1953; **265**: 1111–20.
15. Cholesterol, atherosclerosis and coronary disease in the UK, 1950–2000. In Reynolds LA, Tansey EM, eds. *Wellcome Witnesses to Twentieth Century Medicine* 2006; **27**: 42.
16. McMichael J. Diet and exercise in coronary heart-disease [Letter]. *Lancet* 1974; **1**: 1340–1.

CHAPTER 2

Lipids gain clinical recognition
Lipid research in the 1960s and 1970s

As will soon become apparent, lipids in general and choles-terol in particular were taken very seriously by basic scientists in the latter part of the twentieth century in Britain. In contrast, clinical lipidology was regarded as a minor branch of chemical pathology, and not a subject with which any practising physician would wish to become involved. It remains a subspecialty, but nowadays the importance of some knowledge of lipids in the management and prevention of cardiovascular disease is accepted by most clinicians.

Early British workers

Alistair Frazer, head of the Department of Medical Biochemistry and Pharmacology at the University of Birmingham in the 1950s, can arguably be regarded as the founding father of clinical research on lipids in Britain. His main interests were the mech-anism of lipid absorption and the malabsorption of dietary fat associated with intestinal disorders such as coeliac disease and tropical sprue. He was a large man, and this, together with his scientific pursuits, led to his being known as 'Fats' Frazer. In his introduction to an issue of the *British Medical Bulletin* in 1958 devoted to the metabolism of lipids, Frazer stated: 'Agreement has not been reached on the precise aetiological relationship between blood lipids and atheroma, although few would deny its existence.'[1] As things transpired, he was right on the first count, but not on the second.

One of the more notable contributions to that issue of the *British Medical Bulletin* was a paper on the biosynthesis of choles-terol by Cornforth and Popjak; the former was later to receive the Nobel Prize in Chemistry and a knighthood for his research on that topic. His co-author, George Popjak, was head of the

Medical Research Council (MRC) Experimental Radiopathology
Unit at Hammersmith Hospital at the time, and some thought
he should have shared the Nobel Prize with Cornforth. In 1953,
Popjak's unit was joined by Nicolas (Nick) Myant, who had been
a house physician to both Sir Thomas Lewis (during the war)
and John McMichael (after the war). Subsequently, Myant
embarked on a lifelong career with the MRC, first at University
College Hospital and then at the Hammersmith, where, more
than 50 years later, he still pursues his research as a retired MRC
worker. Myant recalls that Popjak was convinced of the validity
of the lipid hypothesis and considered that understanding
cholesterol synthesis would contribute to the treatment of
coronary heart disease:[2] how right he was.

Myant and familial hypercholesterolaemia

When Popjak left the Hammersmith in 1962, Myant became a
member of the external staff of the MRC. At that stage, his main
research interest was the thyroid gland, including the effect of
thyroxine on cholesterol synthesis and the treatment of thyro-
toxicosis with radioactive iodine (^{131}I). In 1963, he was joined by
Barry Lewis from Cape Town, a contemporary of Bronte-Stewart,
who had previously undertaken research on lipids with Brock in
South Africa and then with Tom Pilkington at St George's
Hospital in London. After Lewis's arrival at Hammersmith,
Myant's research activities became more lipid oriented and
clinical, the latter facilitated by his being given access to four
beds within the hospital. Together they set up an outpatient
lipid clinic, the first in Britain, and began to undertake research
into the regulation of cholesterol metabolism and the treatment
of patients with familial hypercholesterolaemia (FH).

In 1964, Myant and Lewis used manual plasmapheresis on
four occasions to treat a young girl with homozygous FH in a
desperate attempt to lower her cholesterol.[3] Soon afterwards, de
Gennes et al in Paris adopted a similar approach (they termed it
'traitment héroique') in another FH homozygote, who under-
went manual plasmapheresis on more than 40 occasions over a
period of 3 months; this temporarily reduced his cholesterol but
was too onerous to continue permanently.[4] Both these patients
had severe atherosclerosis, and their subsequent deaths from
cardiovascular disease at the ages of 13 and 23 respectively were,
unfortunately, par for the course in those days. Ten years later,
the advent of the continuous flow blood cell separator enabled
online plasma exchange with albumin to be performed with
speed and safety in patients with homozygous FH[5] at the Hammersmith and led to a significant improvement in their longevity.[6]

My own introduction to lipids began in 1963 as a registrar in gastroenterology to Chris (now Sir Christopher) Booth at the Hammersmith when I became involved in research into the absorption of fat-soluble vitamin D, as described elsewhere.[7] To carry out these studies, Chris Booth suggested I should acquire some lipid and radioisotopic expertise in Nick Myant's laboratory, and with Barry Lewis's help I managed to master the rudiments of Folch extraction, thin-layer chromatography, preparative ultracentrifugation and liquid scintillation counting. Lewis later moved to the Department of Chemical Pathology but continued with his research on lipids. Subsequently, he was appointed to the Chair of Chemical Pathology at St Thomas's Hospital, where he built up a research group which included Norman Miller, who, with his brother George, had earlier spotlighted the role of high-density lipoprotein (HDL) cholesterol deficiency as a cardio-vascular risk factor.[8] The St Thomas's group went on to conduct the first randomized angiographic trial in Britain to show the beneficial effects of lowering low-density lipoprotein (LDL) on coronary artery disease.[9]

Myant remained a member of the external staff of the MRC at Hammersmith until 1969, when space became available in the Cyclotron Unit. His group was then reconstituted as the MRC Lipid Metabolism Unit, which I joined in 1975, and which he directed until he retired in 1983 (Figure 2.1). During that period, the main focus of his research was FH, the association of which with coronary disease had first been described by a Norwegian physician, Müller.[10] This disorder recalls Robert

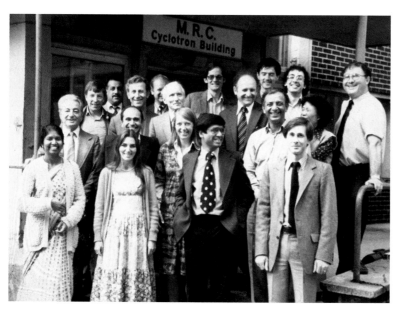

Figure 2.1 *The MRC Lipid Metab-olism Unit in 1983 with its Director, Nick Myant (centre of third row)*

Frost's comment, 'Nature is always hinting at us', the hint in question being that the presence of hypercholesterolaemia from birth onwards results in premature atherosclerosis and cardiovascular disease. The age of onset of the latter is determined by the severity of the hypercholesterolaemia; it occurs in childhood in homozygotes and in adulthood in heterozygotes. Myant was especially interested in the mechanism of the hypercholesterolaemia in FH, and he undertook studies of the turnover of ^{14}C-labelled cholesterol to determine whether increased synthesis or decreased catabolism of cholesterol was responsible, but with inconclusive results.[11]

During the ensuing years, Nick Myant had a major influence on lipid research in Britain and is regarded with affectionate respect by all who worked with him, and by many others besides. His scrupulous approach to scientific research is exemplified by the following excerpt from the Preface to his book on cholesterol, published in 1981:

> It should not be necessary to refer here to the need for balance and objectivity in the sifting of evidence, something that has been taken for granted by the scientific community for about 300 years. Nevertheless, it is a fact that the very word 'cholesterol' tends to arouse emotional reactions that cloud judgement.... The reason for this state of affairs is, of course, the link thought to exist between cholesterol and a disease so serious and widespread that it is difficult not to feel strongly about it.... I see no advantage in adopting an evangelistic approach, since the question will ultimately be settled by the methods of science. It seems to me that those engaged in the current controversy should try to emulate Darwin, one of whose endearing traits was a horror of being unfair to his opponents ... he kept a special notebook for facts that went against his theory because he found that he tended to forget them.[12]

American pioneers

Inherited disorders of lipid metabolism such as FH were also the object of considerable attention during the 1950s and 1960s from Donald (Don) Fredrickson at the US National Institutes of Health (NIH) in Bethesda, Maryland. He joined the staff there in 1953 and published his first paper on lipids the following year. He later recalled attending a symposium in 1957 in New Orleans with Ancel Keys, Alistair ('Fats') Frazer and John Youmans, Dean of Vanderbilt University. The last-named took them to a bar in the French quarter, where they ran up a large bill buying watered-down drinks for the bar girls. Youmans had apparently been a jazz trumpeter in the city in his youth, so he knew the ropes and led them out without paying, pursued by the bartenders and girls.[13]

Fredrickson's research focused on the role of lipoproteins in transporting lipids in plasma and the familial disorders characterized by lipoprotein abnormalities in patients who had been referred to the NIH. In 1961, he and his colleagues were the first to describe an inherited deficiency of HDL characterized by enlarged, orange-coloured tonsils, which they called 'Tangier disease' because the first two patients lived on Tangier Island, which is situated in Chesapeake Bay just off the coast of Virginia. Fredrickson was appointed Director of the National Heart Institute in 1966 and became the Director of the NIH in 1975.

At the beginning of 1967, Fredrickson, Levy and Lees published a multipart paper in the *New England Journal of Medicine*, which described the phenotypic classification of five different types of hyperlipoproteinaemia[14] and thereby revolutionized the attitude of clinicians to lipids. Among those infected with enthusiasm were two young interns, Goldstein and Brown, at the Massachusetts General Hospital (MGH), Boston. (I was a research fellow at the MGH at that time, and I can still recall the excitement generated by that paper.) Joe Goldstein subsequently looked after Fredrickson's patients as a clinical associate at the NIH, and it was this experience which stimulated his interest in FH, an interest he communicated to Mike Brown. Their subsequent scientific collaboration at the University of Texas Southwestern Medical School in Dallas resulted in their discovery of the LDL receptor and the role played by genetic abnormalities of the latter in causing FH,[15] findings which led to their being awarded the Nobel Prize in 1985. Fredrickson's colleague at the NIH, Robert (Bob) Levy, had earlier shown that the fractional rate of turnover of ^{125}I-labelled LDL was reduced in FH patients,[16] implying the existence of an in vivo catabolic defect, and the underlying deficiency of LDL receptors that was responsible was revealed by Goldstein and Brown's in vitro studies.[17]

Another of the interns at the MGH at that time was Antonio (Tony) Gotto, and he, too, came under Fredrickson's aegis at the NIH. He was subsequently invited to establish a lipid research group at Baylor College of Medicine in Houston, and I joined him there in 1972, the year that Goldstein and Brown embarked on their seminal studies in nearby Dallas. The 1970s were halcyon years for clinicians and biochemists interested in lipids, but, as will become apparent later, the relevance of the advances in lipidology to atherosclerosis and coronary disease was disputed by certain cardiologists, who were accused, in a paper at the time, of practising 'paleocardiology', as distinct from 'neocardiology'.[18]

'The climb to base camp'

Fredrickson later summarized the progress which occurred between 1950 and 1975 as a Bethesda-driven 'climb to base camp' that preceded the conjunction of molecular biology with the research done on lipoproteins and dyslipoproteinaemia.[19] His inspiration and leadership during that early phase of exploration were an essential preliminary to the successful scaling of scientific peaks by others, such as Goldstein and Brown. It would be hard to overestimate the influence he exerted on lipid research and research workers throughout the world during that remarkable era of progress. By differentiating between the phenotypes of the various types of lipoprotein disorder, Fredrickson stimulated the search for the pathological mechanisms responsible and thereby set the stage for the discovery of the underlying gene defects.

References

1. Frazer AC. Lipid metabolism: introduction. *Br Med Bull* 1958; **14**: 197–200.
2. Myant NB. Introduction. Cholesterol, atherosclerosis and coronary disease in the UK, 1950–2000. In Reynolds LA, Tansey EM, eds. *Wellcome Witnesses to Twentieth Century Medicine* 2006; **27**: xxiii.
3. Myant NB. Introduction. Cholesterol, atherosclerosis and coronary disease in the UK, 1950–2000. In Reynolds LA, Tansey EM, eds. *Wellcome Witnesses to Twentieth Century Medicine* 2006; **27**: xxiv.
4. De Gennes JL, Touraine R, Maunand B, et al. Homozygous cutaneo-tendinous forms of hypercholesteremic xanthomatosis in an exemplary familial case. Trial of plasmapheresis: an heroic treatment. *Bull Mem Soc Med Hop Paris* 1967; **118**: 1377–1402.
5. Thompson GR, Lowenthal R, Myant NB. Plasma exchange in the management of homozygous familial hypercholesterolaemia. *Lancet* 1975; **1**: 1208–11.
6. Thompson GR, Miller JP, Breslow JL. Improved survival of patients with homozygous familial hypercholesterolaemia treated with plasma exchange. *Br Med J* 1985; **291**: 1671–3.
7. Thompson GR. *Hammersmith Marathon*. London: Royal Society of Medicine Press, 1999.
8. Miller GJ, Miller NE. Plasma-high-density-lipoprotein concentration and development of ischaemic heart-disease. *Lancet* 1975; **1**: 16–20.
9. Watts GF, Lewis B, Brunt JN, et al. Effects on coronary artery disease of lipid-lowering diet, or diet plus cholestyramine in the St Thomas' Atherosclerosis Regression Study (STARS). *Lancet* 1992; **339**: 563–9.

10. Müller C. Angina pectoris in hereditary xanthomatosis. *Arch Intern Med* 1939; **64**: 675–700.
11. Myant NB. The regulation of cholesterol metabolism as related to familial hypercholesterolaemia. *Sci Basis Med Annu Rev* 1970: 230–59.
12. Myant NB. *The Biology of Cholesterol and Related Sterols*. London: Heinemann, 1981.
13. http://profiles.nlm.nih.gov/FF/B/B/L/G/_/ffbblg.txt.
14. Fredrickson DS, Levy RI, Lees RS. Fat transport in lipoproteins – an integrated approach to mechanisms and disorders. *N Engl J Med* 1967; **276**: 34–42, 94–103, 148–56, 215–25, 273–81.
15. Goldstein JL, Brown MS. Familial hypercholesterolemia: identification of a defect in the regulation of 3-hydroxy-3-methylglutaryl coenzyme A reductase activity associated with overproduction of cholesterol. *Proc Natl Acad Sci U S A* 1973; **70**: 2804–8.
16. Langer T, Strober W, Levy RI. The metabolism of low density lipoprotein in familial type II hyperlipoproteinemia. *J Clin Invest* 1972; **51**: 1528–36.
17. Brown MS, Goldstein JL. Familial hypercholesterolemia: defective binding of lipoproteins to cultured fibroblasts associated with impaired regulation of 3-hydroxy-3-methylglutaryl coenzyme A reductase activity. *Proc Natl Acad Sci U S A* 1974; **71**: 788–92.
18. Carruthers M, Taggart P. Paleocardiology and neocardiology. *Am Heart J* 1974; **88**: 1–6.
19. Fredrickson DS. Phenotyping. On reaching base camp (1950–1975). *Circulation* 1993; **87**(Suppl 4): III1–15.

CHAPTER 3

Early setbacks for the lipid hypothesis

First-generation cholesterol-lowering diet and drug trials

Demonstrating an association between serum cholesterol and risk of coronary heart disease is an essential prerequisite of the lipid hypothesis, but evidence that lowering cholesterol reduced the risk was needed to prove that the relationship is one of cause and effect. As stated by the sceptical Sir John McMichael, 'All trials of prophylactic measures in CHD [coronary heart disease] based on hypotheses of causation have to be examined in the prevention of progression of the disorder in known patients at risk with proven clinical manifestations.'[1] In other words, the proof of the pudding is in the eating. And in that context, the results of the early lipid-lowering trials, conducted in the 1960s and 1970s, were more often than not decidedly unpalatable.

Role of diet

The best epidemiological evidence at that time of the relationship between diet, serum cholesterol and coronary heart disease was the Seven Countries Study, conceived by Ancel Keys.[2] This showed correlations, across countries, between the percentage of men with a raised serum cholesterol and the percentage of dietary calories derived from saturated fat. Furthermore, countries with a high intake of saturated fat, such as Finland and the USA, had a higher incidence of coronary heart disease than countries, such as Japan and Greece, where the saturated fat intake was low and raised serum cholesterol was infrequent.

Keys had previously shown that reducing saturated fat intake by a given amount had a cholesterol-lowering effect roughly equivalent to supplementing the diet with twice that amount of polyunsaturated fat. Hence, the early coronary prevention trials utilized either a low-fat diet or a diet enriched in polyunsaturated fat to lower serum cholesterol. Furthermore, as stipulated by McMichael, the trials were undertaken in patients who had sustained a myocardial infarct in the past; that is, they were secondary prevention trials.

Secondary prevention trials

The results of two such trials undertaken in Britain were published in 1965, one of which used corn oil[3] and the other a low-fat diet.[4] Both were negative. A third trial, larger and lasting longer, used soya bean oil, which lowered serum cholesterol by 12%, but, again, had a disappointingly negative outcome.[5] Slightly more encouraging results were seen in diet trials conducted in Europe[6,7] and the USA.[8] These achieved greater decreases in serum cholesterol than the British trials and provided evidence of a possible reduction in coronary events in younger patients.[6,8] But the verdict at this stage in relation to preventing coronary heart disease by dietary change was, at best, case unproven. Consequently, interest shifted towards lowering serum cholesterol by pharmacological means.

In 1963, Oliver reported the lipid-lowering properties of chlorphenoxyisobutyric acid, later known as clofibrate.[9] This compound had been developed by ICI under the trade name Atromid, and it was used in two secondary prevention trials, conducted in Scotland[10] and Newcastle.[11] These trials started in 1964 and lasted for over 5 years, and both showed a significant reduction in mortality and in non-fatal myocardial infarcts in patients with angina receiving clofibrate compared with those on placebo. However, there was no evidence that this was due to the 11–12% reduction in serum cholesterol that was observed. Other possible explanations were the effects of clofibrate in reducing free fatty acids and fibrinogen, and in reducing platelet activity. Although the outcome of these trials must have been encouraging for the cardiologists involved, the results did little to strengthen the case for the lipid hypothesis, the only supportive piece of evidence being that in the Newcastle trial patients with high baseline cholesterol levels had more events than those with lower levels.

These early prevention trials were reviewed by Shaper, another South African immigrant to make a major contribution to cardiovascular research in Britain, who concluded that 'the gain in knowledge for the vast amount of work expended is not very impressive'.[12] One of the limitations of secondary prevention trials is that the outcome is determined more by the extent of myocardial damage consequent on previous infarction than by the severity of the underlying coronary atherosclerosis. On the other hand, because the incidence of myocardial infarction in middle-aged men was only about 1% per year, the sample size of a primary prevention trial would have to be much larger to achieve a conclusive result within 5–10 years.

Primary prevention trials

With these requirements in mind, and with the support of the World Health Organization (WHO), Oliver and Morris and others embarked in 1965 on a double-blind, multicentre trial of primary prevention in over 15 000 men aged 30–59.[13] All subjects were free from coronary heart disease at the outset and were observed for just over 5 years. The treatment group, consisting of over 5000 men whose serum cholesterol was in the top third of the cholesterol distribution, averaging 6.8 mmol/l, received clofibrate 1.6 g/day, and a similarly chosen control group received a placebo. There was also a second control group with serum cholesterol values in the bottom third of the distribution. Serum cholesterol decreased by 9% in the clofibrate group, and this was associated with a 25% decrease in non-fatal myocardial infarcts ($P < 0.05$) compared with the control group with initially comparable cholesterol values. However, the incidence of fatal myocardial infarcts in the two groups was similar, and the crude death rate was actually higher in clofibrate-treated subjects ($P < 0.05$), mainly due to an excess of deaths from diseases involving the liver, biliary system and intestines. Beneficial effects of clofibrate were most obvious in individuals who smoked, who had raised blood pressure, and whose cholesterol decreased the most. The authors concluded that lowering the serum cholesterol level reduced the incidence of coronary heart disease, but that clofibrate had too many disadvantages to be used for this purpose in the general population.

The latter impression was reinforced 2 years later when the WHO investigators published an analysis of over 5 years of in-trial and more than 4 years of follow-up data.[14] This showed that clofibrate-treated subjects had sustained a 25% increase in total mortality, which sounded the death knell for clofibrate and posed difficult questions for adherents of the lipid hypothesis in Britain. The WHO trial undoubtedly raised serious doubts for Michael Oliver (Figure 3.1) about the safety of cholesterol-lowering therapy, doubts which must have influenced his attitude to coronary prevention for many years afterwards.

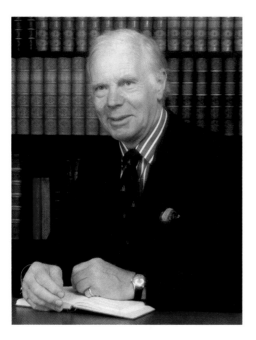

Figure 3.1 *Michael Oliver*

A glimmer of hope for lipid-lowerers came from Norway, with the publication a few years later of the results of the Oslo Trial of Diet and Smoking Intervention.[15] This was a primary prevention trial in over 1200 high-risk men randomized into two groups. Those in the intervention group were given dietary advice and asked to decrease their consumption of tobacco. During the 5-year period of the trial, the intervention group showed a 13% decrease in serum total cholesterol level and a 45% decrease in tobacco consumption compared with the controls. At the end of the trial, the incidence of fatal plus non-fatal myocardial infarction plus sudden death was 45% lower in the intervention group than in the controls, this being significant at the 3% level. It was estimated that 25% of the reduction in risk was due to the change in smoking habits, the remainder being attributed to the decrease in serum cholesterol levels achieved by diet.

Less encouraging were the largely negative results of two other multifactorial risk factor intervention trials, one in the USA[16] and the other in Europe.[17] The latter involved four different countries, one of which was Britain, where, despite advice aimed at reducing serum cholesterol and smoking, no decrease in coronary heart disease was observed.

One of the last of the lipid-lowering trials conducted in the pre-statin era was the Lipid Research Clinics Coronary Primary Prevention Trial (LRC–CPPT), a multicentre, double-blind trial of cholesterol lowering in the primary prevention of coronary heart disease in North America.[18] This involved screening almost 500000 men aged 38–59, of whom 3806 were identified with serum total cholesterol level higher than 6.8 mmol/l, and who were free from overt coronary heart disease. After randomization, both groups were put on a cholesterol-lowering diet; in addition, the test group was given 24 g cholestyramine resin per day, whereas the control subjects received a matching placebo. After 7–10 years, average levels of serum total and low-density lipoprotein (LDL) cholesterol in the cholestyramine group were 8.5% and 12.6% lower, respectively, than those of the placebo group. There was a 19% reduction in deaths from coronary heart disease plus non-fatal myocardial infarcts in the cholestyramine group but no significant difference between the two groups in total mortality.

To ascertain whether the reduction of risk was related to the degree of reduction of hypercholesterolaemia, the 155 men in the cholestyramine-treated group who had sustained a coronary event during the trial were subdivided according to the year when this occurred.[19] The reduction of LDL cholesterol in these individuals was compared with the reduction in those who had remained free from coronary heart disease over the same period. The results suggested that a decrease in serum total cholesterol level of 26% or a decrease in LDL cholesterol level of 35% would halve the risk of developing coronary heart disease in hyper-cholesterolaemic men.

Levy and Fredrickson

The Lipid Research Clinics Program had been established in 1970 and was headed initially by Bob Levy and later by Basil Rifkind, a Glaswegian cardiologist who had recently emigrated to the USA. Levy and colleagues conceived the LRC–CPPT, which took place in 12 centres during the 1970s and was completed during his tenure as Director of the National Heart, Lung and Blood Institute. This was at a time when the entire future of lipid-lowering therapy was in doubt as a result of the negative publicity generated by earlier trials. Hearsay has it that when the results of the LRC–CPPT were being analysed, the statisticians involved were locked in a room at the National Institutes of Health (NIH) and told they would be let out only after they had come to a favourable decision. Eventually, a note came out under the door asking whether a reduction in coronary events which was significant at the 5% level on the basis of a one-tailed *t*-test was acceptable! It was, but only just.

Although there was no decrease in total mortality, this result was sufficient to convince many of the doubters that cholesterol-lowering therapy was effective and thereby ensure its future as a clinical endeavour. For that reason, and many others besides, Bob Levy has earned a place in history alongside his old boss and predecessor at the NIH, Don Fredrickson. At a personal level they were as different as chalk and cheese – Levy was brought up in the Bronx and his direct manner upset some people, whereas Fredrickson's urbane sophistication could charm a bird off a tree. Between them, however, they provided the basis of knowledge upon which the diagnosis and management of dyslipidaemia currently rests. The remarkable decrease in coronary heart disease in the USA since 1980, almost a quarter of which has been attributed to reductions in serum cholesterol,[20] is due in no small part to their efforts in this respect.

References

1. McMichael J. Prevention of coronary heart disease. *Lancet* 1976; **2**: 1350–1.
2. Keys A. Coronary heart disease in seven countries. *Circulation* 1970; **41**(Suppl 1): 1–199.
3. Rose GA, Thomson WB, Williams RT. Corn oil in treatment of ischaemic heart disease. *Br Med J* 1965; **1**: 1531–3.
4. Research Committee. Low-fat diet in myocardial infarction. A controlled trial. *Lancet* 1965; **2**: 501–4.
5. Report of a Research Committee to the Medical Research Council. Controlled trial of soya-bean oil in myocardial infarction. *Lancet* 1968; **2**: 693–9.
6. Leren P. The effect of plasma cholesterol lowering diet in male survivors of myocardial infarction. *Acta Med Scand* 1966; (Suppl 466): 1–92.
7. Miettinen M, Turpeinen O, Karvonen MJ, et al. Effect of cholesterol lowering diet on mortality from coronary heart disease and other causes. *Lancet* 1972; **2**: 835–8.
8. Dayton S, Pearce ML, Goldman H, et al. Controlled trial of a diet high in unsaturated fat for prevention of atherosclerotic complications. *Lancet* 1968; **2**: 1060–2.
9. Oliver MF. Further observations on the effects of Atromid and of ethyl chlorophenoxyisobutyrate on serum lipid levels. *J Atheroscler Res* 1963; **3**: 427–44.
10. Report by a Research Committee of the Scottish Society of Physicians. Ischaemic heart disease: a secondary prevention trial using clofibrate. *Br Med J* 1971; **4**; 775–84.
11. Five-year study by a group of physicians of the Newcastle upon Tyne region. Trial of clofibrate in the treatment of ischaemic heart disease. *Br Med J* 1971; **4**: 767–75.
12. Shaper AG. Primary and secondary prevention trials in coronary heart disease. *Postgrad Med J* 1976; **52**: 464–9.
13. Report from the Committee of Principal Investigators. A co-operative trial in the primary prevention of ischaemic heart disease using clofibrate. *Br Heart J* 1978; **40**: 1069–118.
14. Report of the Committee of Principal Investigators. W.H.O. cooperative trial on primary prevention of ischaemic heart disease using clofibrate to lower serum cholesterol: mortality follow up. *Lancet* 1980; **2**: 379–85.
15. Hjermann I, Velve Byre K, Holme I, Leren P. Effect of diet and smoking intervention on the incidence of coronary heart disease. Report from the Oslo study group of a randomised trial in healthy men. *Lancet* 1981; **2**: 1303–10.
16. Multiple Risk Factor Intervention Trial Group. Multiple Risk Factor Intervention Trial. *JAMA* 1982; **248**: 1465–77.
17. World Health Organization European Collaborative Group. European collaborative trial of multi-factorial prevention of coronary heart disease: final report on the 6 year results. *Lancet* 1986; **1**: 869–72.

18. Lipid Research Clinics Program. The Lipid Research Clinics Coronary Primary Prevention Trial results. I. Reduction in incidence of coronary heart disease. *JAMA* 1984; **251**: 351–64.
19. Lipid Research Clinics Program. The Lipid Research Clinics Coronary Primary Prevention Trial results. II. The relationship of reduction in incidence of coronary heart disease to cholesterol lowering. *JAMA* 1984; **251**: 365–74.
20. Ford ES, Ajani UA, Croft JB, et al. Explaining the decrease in U.S. deaths from coronary disease, 1980–2000. *N Engl J Med* 2007; **356**: 2388–98.

CHAPTER 4

Pure and white but not deadly
John Yudkin's sugar hypothesis

The early 1970s was a period of transition for those working in the lipid field, most of whom were still digesting the advances made by Fredrickson and his colleagues and trying to keep pace with the ever-lengthening alphabet of recently discovered apolipoproteins. In an effort to get to grips with the latter, I spent much of 1972 and 1973 working in Tony Gotto's laboratory in Texas, funded by the Lipid Research Clinics Program.

In the 2 years preceding my move to Houston, Barry Lewis and I had organized postgraduate courses on 'Clinical and biochemical aspects of lipid metabolism' at the Hammersmith. Among our guest speakers were Lars Carlson, Basil Rifkind, Gerry Shaper, Jerry Morris and Michael Oliver. The courses were well attended, and over 30% of the participants came from overseas. Five years later, after Lewis had moved to St Thomas's, Nick Myant and I organized a similar course, on 'Lipoprotein metabolism and its disorders', the change in title illustrating the shift in emphasis from lipids to lipoproteins that had taken place during that time.

In contrast to the rapid advances in knowledge of the structure and function of lipoproteins, early attempts to influence the progression of atherosclerosis and prevent coronary disease by lowering serum cholesterol by diet or drugs were unrewarding, as has already been discussed. The absence of any convincing evidence that lowering cholesterol influences clinical outcome rendered the lipid hypothesis open to criticism and left room for alternative explanations for the rise in coronary mortality since the end of the Second World War. This trend reached its peak in 1970, when the UK was second only to Finland in the world rankings of national coronary mortality rates.

The sugar hypothesis is aired

In the summer of 1974, *The Times* published an article entitled 'Why suspicion falls on sugar as a major cause of heart disease'. The author was John Yudkin, Emeritus Professor of Nutrition at Queen Elizabeth College, University of London, whose work at the time was supported by the National Dairy Council.[1] Yudkin had previously reported that the increase in coronary disease in Britain was proportional to the increase in radio and television licences and he suggested that the evidence linking saturated fat, serum cholesterol and coronary disease was in a similar category, lacking proof of causality. In particular, the lack of evidence from dietary trials that modifying fat intake reduces the risk of coronary heart disease made him conclude that the lipid hypothesis was defunct. Among the alternative explanations he proposed were a lack of roughage or trace elements in the diet, and excess of protein, carbohydrate or sugar.[2]

Consumption of sugar in Britain had increased 25-fold during the past 200 years, and Yudkin cited data showing that a high intake of sucrose could raise serum cholesterol and triglyceride, especially the latter, as well as levels of insulin, cortisol and uric acid, and that it also impaired glucose tolerance and induced a clotting tendency. All these abnormalities were evident in subjects with coronary disease, so he claimed, and he proposed that they reflected a hormonal disturbance brought about by excessive consumption of sucrose. He concluded that eating less sugar would correct the hormonal imbalance and also favourably influence dental disease, diabetes and obesity, whereas altering dietary fat intake, particularly increasing the intake of polyunsaturated fats, would achieve none of these objectives and might have adverse side-effects.

Earlier that year Yudkin had contributed to a report of the Committee on Medical Aspects (COMA) of Food Policy on diet in relation to cardiovascular disease.[3] The majority of the other members of the committee recommended that the amount of total and saturated fat in the UK diet should be reduced to decrease cardiovascular disease and that sucrose consumption should be reduced to decrease obesity. However, in a note of reservation at the end of the report, Yudkin recorded his opinion that the role of dietary fat in causing cardiovascular disease had been exaggerated and that the role of sucrose had been minimized. One of the other members of the committee, JRA Mitchell, was subsequently highly critical of Yudkin, especially his citing as evidence theoretical speculations bearing no proven relationship to the matter under discussion. According to Mitchell, the panel had agreed from the outset that these were to be regarded as 'black box' items, the box being marked 'only to be opened if a link between nutrition and vascular disease is established'.[4]

Yudkin's claims regarding the link between sugar and vascular disease were based on remarkably scanty experimental evidence. In 1964, he and Roddy[5] had shown that the estimated intake of sucrose in 45 men with coronary or peripheral vascular disease was significantly greater than that of 25 controls. On the basis of these results, the authors claimed that the relationship between sucrose and vascular disease was causal and that people taking over 110 g/day were five times more likely to develop myocardial infarction than those taking under 60 g/day. Three years later, following criticisms of the methodology used to estimate sucrose intake, Yudkin and Morland carried out another study, modified so as to minimize any bias in estimating dietary intake, in 20 myocardial infarct survivors and 33 controls, and again found a significantly higher intake of sucrose among the former.[6]

The MRC investigates

In the light of these findings, the Medical Research Council (MRC) convened a working party to investigate the relationship between sugar and vascular disease. Studies were performed in four centres, two in London and two in Scotland. The largest study took place at the Central Middlesex Hospital, where Richard Doll was involved, while the one conducted at the Edinburgh Royal Infirmary was supervised by Michael Oliver. The pooled results of all these studies showed no difference between the sucrose intake of 122 myocardial infarct survivors and 113 controls, leading the working party to conclude, in 1970, 'the evidence in favour of a high sugar intake as a major factor in the development of myocardial infarction is extremely slender.'[7]

The media debate

Despite the working party's conclusion, Yudkin persevered in his beliefs, which he not only published in a book[8] but, as noted earlier, he also reiterated 4 years later in *The Times*. I managed to persuade the newspaper to allow me to rebut Yudkin's claims and put the case for saturated fat, rather than sucrose, being the dietary cause of cardiovascular disease. My article was entitled 'Beware sweet reason in the search for causes of heart disease',[9] and it concluded that the evidence linking sucrose and cardio-vascular disease was largely circumstantial, similar to that linking television sets and heart attacks, whereas the evidence that saturated fat was harmful was much stronger.

The Times articles caught the eye of a producer at the BBC, who arranged for a debate to take place at the Royal Institution in September 1974, which was recorded and transmitted subsequently in the *Controversy* series on television. The motion to be debated was 'The dietary cause of heart disease is sugar, not fat', proposed by John Yudkin and opposed by Don Fredrickson (Figure 4.1), assisted by Peter Taggart and myself, with Sir George Porter, Nobel laureate in chemistry, in the chair. Peter Taggart was a cardiologist at the Middlesex Hospital whose interest in lipids stemmed from his observation that racing drivers can develop stress-induced hyperlipidaemia. Despite being outnumbered, Yudkin put up a stiff resistance and kept bouncing back like a punchball despite repeated verbal knockdowns. After the debate was over, Don Fredrickson and I had dinner together in a nearby restaurant. At that stage he was President of the Institute of Medicine of the National Academy of Sciences in Washington and about to become Director of the National Institutes of Health (NIH), although one would never have guessed it from his relaxed and unassuming manner. In the latter role, he soon became involved in another controversy, over recombinant DNA research, and was instrumental in getting this legitimized in the face of considerable opposition. He was a man of great charm and wit, the exception which proves the rule that 'nice guys finish last!'

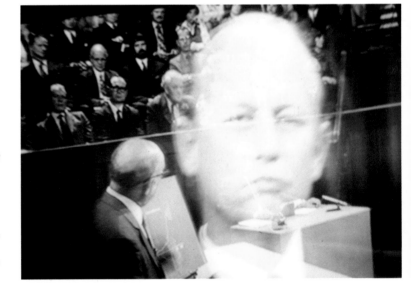

Figure 4.1 *Double take of John Yudkin (left) presenting the case for his sugar hypothesis and Don Fredrickson (right) opposing it during a televised debate at the Royal Institution in 1974*

Yudkin in retrospect

The sucrose hypothesis soon faded away, although the biochemical abnormalities which Yudkin attributed to excess sugar consumption have now become recognized as being part of the metabolic syndrome. The latter is an accompaniment of the central obesity which is becoming increasingly common nowadays as a result of excessive caloric intake, especially when derived from rapidly absorbed carbohydrate. Individuals with the metabolic syndrome have an increased liability to develop coronary heart disease, so in this respect Yudkin was right. Where he erred was in overemphasizing the role of sucrose, despite the evidence against it, and in disregarding the role of saturated fat, despite the evidence for it. Official acceptance of his views could have had unforeseen consequences for the population approach to prevention of coronary heart disease in Britain, but, happily, this did not occur. The only reference to sugar in the recommendations from COMA 10 years later regarding cardiovascular prevention was that the intake of sucrose, glucose and fructose should not increase any further.[10]

Yudkin's views on diet and heart disease must have been music to the ears of the National Dairy Council. The late Keith Ball, one of the earliest advocates of dietary change to prevent coronary disease, criticized the massive advertising campaign conducted by the Butter Information Council and the National Dairy Council to persuade doctors and the public to disregard official advice to reduce saturated fat intake.[11] He claimed that general practitioners had been circulated with the names of experts who disagreed with the views expressed by official bodies such as COMA, and he questioned the ethics of such promotional activities. Yudkin himself, of course, had openly dissociated himself from COMA's views on fat intake while he was a member of the committee in 1974.[3]

John Yudkin died in 1995 and will be remembered not just for his unorthodox views on sucrose but also as the holder of the first Chair of Nutrition in the UK, established at Queen Elizabeth College, which later honoured him by making him a Fellow. He was highly regarded in nutrition circles and in later life developed a keen interest in the history and social effects of food. His scientific heritage is manifest in the shape of his son, a biochemist at Oxford, and also his nephew and namesake, a diabetologist, who, like him, is involved in research into the role of insulin in atherosclerosis.[12]

References

1. Yudkin J. Why suspicion falls on sugar as a major cause of heart disease. *The Times* 1974; 11 July, p 16.
2. Yudkin J. Sucrose and cardiovascular disease. *Proc Nutr Soc* 1972; **31**: 331–7.
3. Department of Health and Social Security. *Diet and Coronary Heart Disease: Report of the Advisory Panel of the Committee on Medical Aspects of Food Policy (Nutrition) on Diet in Relation to Cardiovascular and Cerebrovascular Disease.* London: HMSO, 1974 (Report on Health and Social Subjects, no. 7).
4. Mitchell JRA. Diet and coronary heart disease – a British point of view. *Adv Exp Med Biol* 1977; **82**: 823–7.
5. Yudkin J, Roddy J. Levels of dietary sucrose in patients with occlusive atherosclerotic disease. *Lancet* 1964; **2**: 6–8.
6. Yudkin J, Morland J. Sugar intake and myocardial infarction. *Am J Clin Nutr* 1967; **20**: 503–6.
7. Dietary sugar intake in men with myocardial infarction. Report to the Medical Research Council by its working party on the relationship between dietary sugar intake and arterial disease. *Lancet* 1970; **2**: 1265–71.
8. Yudkin J. *Pure, White and Deadly: The Problem of Sugar.* London: Davis-Poynter, 1972.
9. Thompson GR. Beware sweet reason in the search for causes of heart disease. *The Times* 1974; 31 July, p 16.
10. Department of Health and Social Security. *Diet and Cardiovascular Disease: Report of the Panel on Diet in Relation to Cardiovascular Disease, Committee on Medical Aspects of Food Policy.* London: HMSO, 1984 (Report on Health and Social Subjects, no. 28).
11. Ball K. Prevention of coronary heart-disease. *Lancet* 1979; **2**: 1182.
12. Cholesterol, atherosclerosis and coronary disease in the UK, 1950–2000. In Reynolds LA, Tansey EM, eds. *Wellcome Witnesses to Twentieth Century Medicine* 2006; **27**: 51–3.

CHAPTER 5

The Leader of the Opposition
Sir John McMichael's anti-cholesterol campaign

Chapter summary

- Criticism of official advice

- The European Society for Clinical Investigation debate

- 'Fats and atheroma: an inquest'

- Role of the Royal College of Physicians

- McMichael and the Hammersmith

Sir John McMichael was once described as the greatest clinical scientist of his generation.[1] He directed the Department of Medicine at the Hammersmith from 1946 to 1966, and to those who worked under him he was an Olympian figure akin to 'M' in the James Bond films, evoking in equal measure respect, admiration and affection. He himself attributed the success of the department to the inspired choice of staff made by his predecessor, Francis Frazer, in pre-war years, when the Postgraduate Medical School was founded. These included Paul Wood, Peter Sharpey-Shafer and many other outstanding clinical research workers, including McMichael himself. After the war, however, McMichael's ability to create an atmosphere of enthusiasm, constructive criticism and cooperation was such that the best young research workers were attracted by the reputations of the people working there, and this earned worldwide recognition of the Hammersmith as the best place for postgraduate medical training in the Commonwealth.[2] Many of those he had appointed went on to become professors elsewhere, such as Dame Sheila Sherlock at the Royal Free Hospital and Malcolm Milne at the Westminster Hospital, both of whom became Fellows of the Royal Society. Members of staff and postgraduates who attended the weekly staff round that McMichael chaired with genial authority on Wednesday mornings will recall his gentle handling of young presenters of cases, which could be a nerve-wracking occasion for the uninitiated. This attitude was epitomized by his comment that 'we must have the young upon our shoulders, not trample them under our feet'.[1]

Following his departure from the Hammersmith in 1966, McMichael became Director of the British Postgraduate Medical Federation and continued to influence postgraduate medical training for several years (Figure 5.1). However, under his successor, Chris Booth, his old department changed the direction of its research from the physiological studies he had espoused, and instead focused on investigating mechanisms of disease by biochemical and immunological techniques.

Numerous honours and awards were bestowed upon McMichael, including Fellowship of the Royal Society and a knighthood. In 1975, he gave the Harveian Oration at the Royal College of Physicians, entitled 'A transition in cardiology: the Mackenzie–Lewis era'.[3] During his discourse, he commented, 'Resistance to change is far from unknown among great

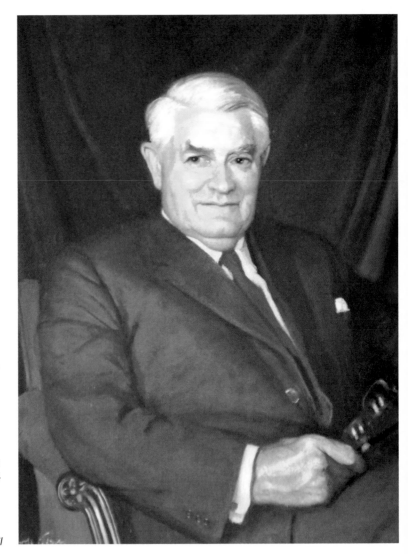

Figure 5.1 *Portrait of Sir John McMichael in the board room of the old Royal Post-graduate Medical School (reproduced with permission from Professor G Screaton, Dean of the Hammersmith Campus, Imperial College). Sir William Hutchison (1968), oil*

scientists', and he exemplified this by Virchow's rejection of Koch's pioneering work. He went on to point out that Mackenzie and Lewis's 'obstinate Celtic temperaments caused them to defend their view' despite overwhelming evidence to the contrary. Ironically, both statements were prophetic of his own attitude to the lipid hypothesis in subsequent years.

Criticism of official advice

In 1973, 3 years after he retired from the British Postgraduate Medical Federation and long after his departure from the Hammersmith, McMichael resumed hostilities with those who believed that diet and exercise play a role in the aetiology of coronary heart disease. In the first of several letters to *The Lancet* from his house in North Square, Hampstead, he criticized the International Society of Cardiology for stating that an increased intake of cholesterol and fat is a prerequisite for the development of atherosclerosis, and once again took issue with Jerry Morris's data showing that exercise has a protective effect.[4] With some reluctance, since I was working in the department he had once directed and where he had given me my first job 11 years previously, I rebutted McMichael's arguments and suggested that cardiologists and those involved in research into atherosclerosis should start a constructive dialogue,[5] a sentiment which fell on deaf ears.

Two years later, McMichael returned to the fray to criticize the recommendations of a joint working party of the Royal College of Physicians and the British Cardiac Society on the prevention of coronary disease, which endorsed the policy of reducing saturated fat intake to lower serum cholesterol.[6] He reiterated his conviction that this measure would have little effect on the incidence of coronary disease and concluded that 'it is better to trust to luck than to foster neurosis by pretence that we can save lives by interfering with life habits'. The chairman of the joint working party, Gerry Shaper, responded that the measures recommended in the report had a reasonable hope of conferring benefit, and none had a cost that approached the cost of inaction.[7] McMichael was unimpressed and again criticized the report for its simplistic dietetic advice and the manner in which its views were publicized by the Department of Health, which had sent a copy to every doctor.[8] Further support for the report came from John Goodwin, who had been a member of McMichael's department from its early days. He had instigated the joint working party when he was President of the British Cardiac Society, and he defended the advice it gave to the medical profession aimed at preventing coronary disease, while accepting that knowledge on this topic was incomplete.[9]

McMichael next turned his attention to the recently published results of the Whitehall Study by Rose and his colleagues and questioned whether the correlation of raised cholesterol with coronary risk in patients with angina or an abnormal electro-cardiogram (ECG) might be a consequence of myocardial ischaemia rather than a cause, as Paul Wood had suggested many years before. He also queried these authors' advocacy of the need for further prevention trials.[10] Geoffrey Rose, an outstanding epidemiologist, and his colleagues tactfully pointed out that McMichael's conclusions were based on a misinterpre-tation of their findings, and suggested that the cost of prevention trials was small compared with that of failing to detect the benefits of prevention or the mistaken adoption of ineffective policies.[11]

The European Society for Clinical Investigation debate

Many of McMichael's criticisms pertaining to lipids and epidemi-ology were scientifically rather naive, but his past achievements and considerable reputation lent credence to his arguments and ensured that they were well publicized. The chance to put them to the test came in 1977, when the European Society for Clinical Investigation held a 'Controversy in medicine' debate at its annual meeting in Rotterdam. The motion to be debated was 'That modification of serum lipids by dietary and/or other means will influence the incidence of, or mortality from, coronary heart disease'. In favour of the motion were Lars Carlson from Stockholm, Shlomo Eisenberg from Jerusalem, and I. Carlson was the leading clinical lipidologist in Europe at the time while Eisenberg had established a major reputation as a result of the research on lipoprotein turnover he had carried out with Levy at the US National Institutes of Health (NIH). Against the motion were Sir John McMichael and Professors Paul Astrup and Christian Crone, both from Copenhagen. The debate was chaired by Hermon Dowling, who was Secretary of the European Society at that time.

The proponents of the motion put forward a tripartite case for there being a causal association between hyperlipidaemia and coronary disease and postulated that reversal of the former would reduce the incidence of the latter. This was based on three lines of scientific evidence, epidemiological, experimental and clinical, presented in an orthodox manner. The case against the motion was put irresistibly by Christian Crone, who showed two slides. The first was a photograph of a sleek, well groomed rat, which, he said, had been fed on butter from birth, while the second showed a malnourished rodent with dull, moulting fur, which, he claimed, had been fed on corn oil throughout its life. The audience dissolved into laughter, and Crone's debating ploy ensured that the motion was lost! McMichael was delighted at the outcome, but Lars Carlson was very upset by what he regarded as the comic antics of the opposition.

'Fats and atheroma: an inquest'

As mentioned earlier, 1978 saw the publication of the results of the World Health Organization's trial of clofibrate, which showed an increase in non-cardiovascular causes of death in those on the drug. McMichael was not slow to capitalize on this finding, and in January 1979 he published a paper in the *British Medical Journal* entitled 'Fats and atheroma: an inquest'.[12] In this, he alluded to the negative results of the early diet trials as casting doubt on the role of cholesterol in atherosclerosis, and he pointed out the potential dangers of lowering blood levels by polyunsaturated fats and clofibrate, namely cancer of the colon and gallstones, respectively. He concluded that official medical endorsement of these cholesterol-reducing measures should be withdrawn. In a similar paper published later that year, he characterized the campaign to substitute polyunsaturated for saturated fats as a 'quite unwarranted extension of hope over experience'.[13]

Taking a leaf out of McMichael's tactics in the Rotterdam debate and satirizing his earlier use of the inquest theme, I sent a letter to the editor of the *Acta Medica Scandinavica* which paraphrased Mark Antony's funeral oration in *Julius Caesar*.[14] This commenced:

> Friends, clinicians, colleagues, lend me your eyes;
> I come to bury the Lipid Hypothesis, not to praise it.

And it ended:

> My heart is in the coffin there with the Lipid Hypothesis,
> And atheroma must regress before it come back to life.

A more serious and reasoned response came from Jim Mann, yet another South African immigrant to Oxford, who systematically rebutted each of McMichael's arguments against the lipid hypothesis and put the case for dietary change.[15] However, it was going to take more than a spoof on Shakespeare and Mann's retrial of the 'negative evidence' to stop Sir John McMichael in his tracks, although from then on his campaign became more political.

Role of the Royal College of Physicians

In 1979, JRA Mitchell, of whom more anon, and McMichael published a letter together in the *Journal of the Royal College of Physicians*, suggesting that the College should withdraw its support for the dietetic recommendations put forward 3 years previously by its joint working party with the British Cardiac Society.[16] McMichael raised the matter in the Comitia of the College, and it was then referred to the Council of the College, which, under the enlightened presidency of Sir Douglas Black, declined to reopen the issue. McMichael was not to be silenced, however, and raised the issue again several times in 1980. Eventually, the College agreed to undertake a further report on the prevention of coronary heart disease but only after the benefits and risks of polyunsaturated fats had been considered by a WHO-sponsored international meeting of cardiologists in 1982. This decision did not placate McMichael, who expressed his displeasure in the Comitia at its January meeting that year.

McMichael and the Hammersmith

In 1985, a special staff round was held at Hammersmith to commemorate Sir John McMichael's eightieth birthday. Sadly, he had by then sustained a severe stroke and was confined to a wheelchair. I presented one of the cases, a patient with severe hyperlipidaemia who had responded well to lipid-lowering therapy. Sir John nodded and smiled benignly, but his aphasia made it impossible to know whether he had changed his mind about cholesterol. It seemed improbable but not impossible, for in his Harveian Oration he had quoted a passage from William Harvey's *De Motu Cordis*: 'Studious good and honest men do not think it degrading to alter their view if truth and a public demonstration so persuade them or regard it as dishonest to desert errors.'

After he died in 1993, a service of thanksgiving was held for him at St Columba's Church of Scotland in London. It was packed with Hammersmith staff, past and present, united in paying tribute to a great man. As Chris Booth said in his obituary, McMichael had created a clinical research environment, unique in Britain at that time, of free discussion and debate in which all, at whatever level of seniority, might join.[1] His opposition to the lipid hypothesis may in part have reflected an ageing man's reaction against the need to acquire sufficient biochemical knowledge to comprehend it fully. Whether or not that was so, the vigour with which he contested its validity helped ensure that proof of the hypothesis, when it eventually came, was based on the hard evidence he had long demanded. Although the errors that men publish live after them, the good that John McMichael did, especially for the Hammersmith, has also survived and, despite Shakespeare, was not interred with his bones.

References

1. Booth C. Sir John McMichael [Obituary]. *Lancet* 1993; **341**: 686.
2. Farewell at Hammersmith. *Br Med J* 1966; **2**: 320.
3. McMichael J. *A Transition in Cardiology: The Mackenzie–Lewis Era. The Harveian Oration of 1975*. London: Royal College of Physicians, 1976.
4. McMichael J. Diet and exercise in coronary heart-disease [Letter]. *Lancet* 1974; **1**: 1340–1.
5. Thompson G. Diet and coronary heart-disease [Letter]. *Lancet* 1974; **2**: 102.
6. McMichael J. Prevention of coronary heart-disease [Letter]. *Lancet* 1976; **2**: 569.
7. Shaper G. Prevention of coronary heart-disease [Letter]. *Lancet* 1976; **2**: 1203–4.
8. McMichael J. Prevention of coronary heart-disease. *Lancet* 1976; **2**: 1350–1.
9. Goodwin JF. Preventing coronary heart-disease [Letter]. *Lancet* 1977; **1**: 302.
10. McMichael J. Risk factors in coronary heart-disease [Letter]. *Lancet* 1977; **1**: 304.
11. Rose G, Reid DD, McCartney P. Risk factors in coronary heart-disease [Letter]. *Lancet* 1977; **1**: 304.
12. McMichael J. Fats and atheroma: an inquest. *Br Med J* 1979; **1**: 173–5.
13. McMichael J. Fats and arterial disease. *Am Heart J* 1979; **98**: 409–12.
14. Thompson G. The lipid hypothesis [Letter]. *Acta Med Scand* 1980; **208**: 341–2.
15. Mann JI. Fats and atheroma: a retrial. *Br Med J* 1979; **1**: 732–4.
16. Mitchell JRA, McMichael J. Letter to the editor. *J R Coll Physicians Lond* 1979; **13**: 73–4.

CHAPTER 6

Should every cow carry a government health warning?
Tony Mitchell, the 'Abominable No Man'

One of the keenest minds and sharpest tongues among critics of the lipid hypothesis belonged to JRA (Tony) Mitchell, the foundation Professor of Medicine at Nottingham University from 1967 until his retirement in 1990. He died the following year from a pulmonary embolus, which was ironic in that clotting was one of his main scientific interests. His early research was carried out in the department of the Regius Professor of Medicine at Oxford, where he and Colin Schwartz studied the pathology of atherosclerosis. In the book they published on the subject, they proposed that turbulent blood flow at sites of arterial branching caused platelets to coalesce and form mural thrombi, resulting in the formation of raised plaques on the arterial intima.[1] This concept was in keeping with Duguid's thrombogenic theory of atherogenesis but contrary to the lipid hypothesis, the validity of which Mitchell constantly questioned. From the mid-1960s onwards, in collaboration with John Hampton, he turned his attention to platelet structure and function, initially in Oxford and then in Nottingham. This led them to study factors influencing platelet behaviour and to undertake clinical trials with anti-platelet drugs in patients with myocardial infarction.

The COMA reports

Tony Mitchell was a member of the first Committee on the Medical Aspects (COMA) of Food Policy on diet and coronary heart disease, which published its recommendations in 1974.[2] Other members of the committee included Oliver, Morris and Yudkin, and Mitchell later gave a revealing account of the manner in which its deliberations were conducted.[3] He described the agreed brief as being to establish whether there was a link between nutrition and cardiovascular disease and, if there was, to determine whether modifying the identified risk factor conferred benefit on the individual or community. After many meetings and draft reports, the committee was able to agree on certain conclusions. These were that ischaemic heart disease was multifactorial in origin and that some of the factors involved were dietary in nature, but that no single one was predominantly responsible. The committee also agreed that changes in diet could reduce serum lipids but that there was no certainty that their reduction would decrease susceptibility to heart disease. The majority of members of the panel accepted the evidence that the death rate from ischaemic heart disease correlated with the saturated fat content of the diet and therefore recommended that the amount of saturated fat in the diet should be reduced. A minority of the members disagreed with this conclusion and felt that this recommendation went beyond the evidence available. However, apart from Yudkin, whose dissent has already been noted, they agreed to support the corporate viewpoint, albeit reluctantly as far as Mitchell was concerned; he undoubtedly belonged to the minority camp on this issue.

In 1984, a second COMA report was published on diet in relation to cardiovascular disease.[4] Tony Mitchell and Michael Oliver were again members of the committee, but it now had several newcomers, including Jim Mann, Geoffrey Rose and Nick Myant. On this occasion the recommendations regarding the need to reduce the saturated fat content of the diet and to increase its ratio of polyunsaturated to saturated fat were far more specific than those made 10 years previously. Nine of the 10 members of the panel concluded that the incidence of coronary heart disease would be reduced by such measures, although they acknowledged that the evidence fell short of proof. The tenth member, who was not named but was undoubtedly Mitchell,[5] believed that the evidence was insufficient to support that conclusion but considered that reducing dietary fat intake might help prevent obesity.

Rejection of the lipid hypothesis

Mitchell amplified his doubts in an editorial review published the same year as the second COMA report.[6] He prefaced it by quoting HL Mencken: 'There's always an easy solution to every human problem – neat, plausible and wrong'. He went on to question which of the beliefs about diet and coronary disease then current would not only be discarded but also derided by the year 2000. He listed them as follows:

- Coronary heart disease is caused by atherosclerosis.
- Atherosclerotic plaques are cholesterol deposits in artery walls.
- Atherosclerosis can be produced in animals by lipid feeding.
- A high serum cholesterol is a risk marker for coronary disease.
- Dietary lipids determine serum cholesterol.

He went on to point out that if these statements were true two further ones followed:

- Dietary lipids cause coronary heart disease.
- Dietary modifications will prevent coronary heart disease.

Mitchell then put his head on the block by stating that, as far as he was concerned, most of these beliefs were untrue or irrelevant. With the benefit of hindsight it is apparent that he was wrong on virtually every count, although this was not so obvious at the time, especially regarding the last statement, in that the evidence from diet trials was at best equivocal.

Mitchell's approach to prevention in the clinic was to tell his patients to stop smoking but to say nothing on issues such as diet. He attributed to Oliver a similarly cautious approach, which led them, he said, to be labelled 'the abominable no-men' by 'cholesterol evangelists'. His own attitude to the latter was equally pejorative. For example, the title of one of his lectures was 'Should every cow carry a government health warning?',[7] while his publications had titles such as 'Diet and arterial disease – the myths and the realities'[8] and 'What constitutes evidence on the dietary prevention of coronary heart disease? Cosy beliefs or harsh facts?'[6] He ended the latter editorial as he had started it, by quoting HL Mencken: 'The most costly of all follies is to believe passionately in the palpably-not-true'. Or is it even more costly to passionately deny, as he did, what later turns out to be true?

Influential cardiologists

During the late 1970s and early 1980s, McMichael and Mitchell voiced their opposition to the lipid hypothesis in unequivocal terms, whereas Oliver adopted a more ambivalent attitude. For example, in an editorial in 1976, he stated, 'the view that raised plasma cholesterol is per se a cause of coronary heart disease is untenable', but then went on to encourage people to reduce their saturated fat intake so as to reduce their risk of coronary heart disease, while omitting to mention that this would result in a decrease in plasma cholesterol.[9] All three of these men were influential cardiologists and their views undoubtedly affected clinical attitudes among their peers. As recounted elsewhere, the therapeutic nihilism they seemingly encouraged was exemplified by a post-coronary artery bypass patient who was referred by his general practitioner to a cardiologist at a teaching hospital for advice regarding control of his severe hyperlipidaemia. The cardiologist stopped the patient's lipid-lowering drugs and told him to forget about his cholesterol and try to live a normal life. Thankfully, neither the general practitioner nor the patient was satisfied with this advice, which, if put into practice, could have had disastrous consequences.[10]

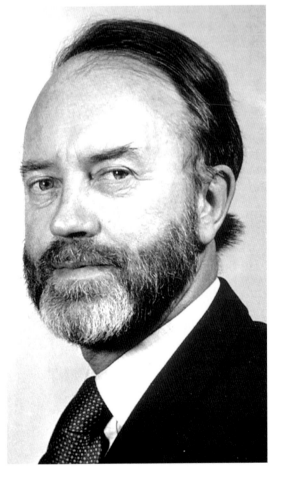

Mitchell maintained his sceptical attitude to the evidence relating to the prevention of coronary disease right up until his retirement in 1990. By then, the results of the early lipid-lowering drug trials were available, including the Lipid Research Clinics Coronary Primary Prevention Trial, which he dismissed as an extravagant waste of money.[11] Like McMichael, he was consistent in his demand for unequivocal proof and, like him, too, he died before it became available.

Despite his 'Dr No' image among supporters of the lipid hypothesis, Tony Mitchell had many positive qualities and was regarded as the major architect of Nottingham's success as a medical school and centre of scientific excellence[7] (Figure 6.1). At one stage, there was a move to persuade him to stand for the presidency of the Royal College

Figure 6.1 *Tony Mitchell (photograph by courtesy of Professor John Hampton)*

of Physicians, but he refused on the grounds that becoming the President would force him to change himself more than he could change the College. His strongly held principles meant that he was unwilling to compromise with National Health Service reforms during the 1980s, and this led him to take early retirement. He was an excellent speaker, discussant and chairman and filled the latter role with distinction for several years in the Atherosclerosis Discussion Group (ADG), which subsequently became the British Atherosclerosis Society (BAS).

The Atherosclerosis Discussion Group

The origins of the ADG go back to 1957, when Michael Oliver, working in Edinburgh, wrote to John French at the Dunn School of Pathology in Oxford, expressing concern that there was no organization in Britain interested in the relationship of lipid metabolism, blood flow and platelets to experimental atherosclerosis. French invited Oliver to come to Oxford to meet his boss, Sir Howard Florey, who, having won the Nobel Prize for his work on penicillin, had now become interested in vascular pathology. At their meeting Florey told French to make a list of those working in the field of atherosclerosis and asked Oliver to raise enough money to hold an inaugural meeting. With the help of Dr 'Cuth' Cuthbertson at Glaxo, Oliver raised the required £250 and French produced a list of people to invite. Florey objected to three on French's list, so more were added, and the first meeting of the new group, comprising 27 members, was held in the autumn of 1958 at the old Medical Research Council headquarters in London, the topic being 'Interrelationships of dietary fat, blood lipids and atherosclerosis'. Lord Florey, as he became, was the first Chairman and Michael Oliver the first Secretary of the ADG, later succeeded by John French. Florey stipulated that there must be an equal time allocated for discussion as for presentation, hence the name Atherosclerosis Discussion Group.

The ADG initially consisted mainly of pathologists plus a few biochemists, cardiologists and people interested in lipid metabolism and blood coagulation. Its membership was limited to 50 and meetings were held twice a year, in the spring and the autumn, initially at the Ciba Foundation in London or at one of the Oxford colleges. In later years, the spring meetings were always held in Oxford, thanks to John Hampton, who, while Secretary of the ADG, persuaded Hugh Sinclair, his old tutor at Magdalen College, to play host there. The autumn ones were then held at Jesus College, Cambridge, where Austin Gresham, the Professor of Pathology, was a Fellow.

The meetings lived up to the group's name, and discussion took up as much if not more time than the presentation of data. The facilities were far from luxurious, the heating being non-existent at Magdalen, and the projection equipment was primitive. Despite this, the multidisciplinary mix of the members and their guests in cramped surroundings resulted in stimulating, close-quarter exchanges between people with opposing views. Tony Mitchell was in his element on these occasions, although he had to exercise considerable self-restraint when he was Chairman. Afterwards protagonists and antagonists chatted amicably over a glass or two of sherry before dining in the hall of the college where the meeting was being held.

In 1975, only three of the 47 members were women, two of whom were pathologists, namely Helen Payling Wright, one of the founder members, and Elspeth Smith, also a founder member and the first to show a relationship between the concentration of LDL in the plasma and the arterial wall.[12] The third was the geneticist Joan Slack, best known for quantifying the risk of coronary disease in familial hypercholesterolaemia. The gender imbalance persisted and Anne Soutar has recalled how few women there still were when she was elected to the ADG, many years later.[13] Yet, despite its elitist nature and distinguished membership, the group as a whole failed to influence medical opinion in Britain regarding the cholesterol controversy as much as it might have done. This may have been because the views of its members on the matter were divided, although there were some, such as Mitchell and Oliver, who were certainly not shy of voicing their opinions in public.

Inevitably, the ADG lost some of its intimacy when it expanded and became the BAS in 1998. However, the emphasis on time for discussion has been preserved, as has the tradition of alternating meetings between Oxford and Cambridge. John French died in 1970, and his influence on the field of atherosclerosis research is commemorated with the John French Memorial Lecture, which is given annually at the spring meeting. French's remarkable insight into the pathology of atherosclerosis is illustrated by the observation he made almost 50 years ago that the lipid composition of the tissue fluid was responsible for the overall severity of tissue changes, whereas the main determinant of clinical events was thrombosis.[14] In an analogous manner, the Hugh Sinclair Memorial Lecture is given at each autumn meeting in recognition of Sinclair's pioneering work on the nutritional aspects of atherosclerosis. Much of what the ADG used to debate with such energy is now old hat, and the emphasis has shifted to topics such as the cell biology of the arterial wall and the role of nuclear receptors in atherosclerosis.

Nevertheless, the BAS continues to offer a means of communication between clinicians and basic scientists doing research on various aspects of atherosclerosis, and thereby perpetuates the aims and objectives of its founders 50 years ago.

References

1. Mitchell JRA, Schwartz CJ. *Arterial Disease*. Oxford: Blackwell Scientific, 1965.
2. Department of Health and Social Security. *Diet and Coronary Heart Disease: Report of the Advisory Panel of the Committee on Medical Aspects of Food Policy (Nutrition) on Diet in Relation to Cardiovascular and Cerebrovascular Disease*. London: HMSO, 1974 (Report on Health and Social Subjects, no. 7).
3. Mitchell JRA. Diet and coronary heart disease – a British point of view. *Adv Exp Med Biol* 1977; **82**: 823–7.
4. Department of Health and Social Security. *Diet and Cardiovascular Disease: Report of the Panel on Diet in Relation to Cardiovascular Disease, Committee on Medical Aspects of Food Policy*. London: HMSO, 1984 (Report on Health and Social Subjects, no. 28).
5. Sanders TAB. Cholesterol, atherosclerosis and coronary disease in the UK, 1950–2000. In Reynolds LA, Tansey EM, eds. *Wellcome Witnesses to Twentieth Century Medicine* 2006; **27**: 62.
6. Mitchell JRA. What constitutes evidence on the dietary prevention of coronary heart disease? Cosy beliefs or harsh facts? *Int J Cardiol* 1984; **5**: 287–98.
7. Obituary. Mitchell JRA. *Br Med J* 1991; **302**: 843.
8. Mitchell JRA. Diet and arterial disease – the myths and the realities. *Proc Nutr Soc* 1985; **44**: 363–70.
9. Oliver M. Dietary cholesterol, plasma cholesterol and coronary heart disease. *Br Heart J* 1976; **38**: 214–18.
10. Thompson GR. Cholesterol, atherosclerosis and coronary disease in the UK, 1950–2000. In Reynolds LA, Tansey EM, eds. *Wellcome Witnesses to Twentieth Century Medicine* 2006; **27**: 11.
11. Mitchell JRA. What do we gain by modifying risk factors for coronary disease? *Schweiz Med Wochenschr* 1990; **120**: 359–64.
12. Smith EB, Slater RS. Relationship between low-density lipoprotein in aortic intima and serum-lipid levels. *Lancet* 1972; **1**: 463–9.
13. Soutar AK. Cholesterol, atherosclerosis and coronary disease in the UK, 1950–2000. In Reynolds LA, Tansey EM, eds. *Wellcome Witnesses to Twentieth Century Medicine* 2006; **27**: 12.
14. French J. 17: Atherosclerosis. In Florey H, ed. *General Pathology* (2nd edn). London: Lloyd-Luke (Medical Books) Ltd, 1958: 351–77.

CHAPTER 7

'Wonder drug that zaps cholesterol'
The discovery and development of statins

The beginning of the end of the controversy over the lipid hypothesis came in 1971, although no one could have forecast this at the time. That was the year when Akira Endo, a Japanese microbiologist working for the pharmaceutical company Sankyo, started searching for microbial metabolites that would inhibit hydroxymethylglutaryl co-enzyme A (HMG CoA) reductase, the key enzyme of cholesterol biosynthesis. His hopes that this would provide a novel means of lowering plasma cholesterol were vindicated when, after testing more than 6000 microbial strains, he and his colleagues isolated a potent inhibitor of HMG CoA reductase from *Penicillium citrinum*, which lowered serum cholesterol in experimental animals.[1,2] Initially known as compactin (ML-236B), this compound was later called mevastatin and became the first HMG CoA reductase inhibitor, or statin, to be used in humans.

Akira Endo

Endo was born in 1933 in Higashiyuri, Japan, where his family farmed. In 1953, he entered the School of Agriculture at Tohoku University, Sendai, and studied biotechnology, graduating in 1957. Immediately after getting his degree, he joined the Sankyo Company in Tokyo. His first project as a member of the applied microbiology group was to develop an enzyme preparation that could be used to hydrolyse pectins contaminating wines and ciders. He succeeded in purifying a new pectinase, and for this work he was awarded his PhD by Tohoku University in 1966. For the next 2 years he did postdoctoral studies in the Department of Molecular Biology at the Albert Einstein College of Medicine in New York, working on a phospholipid-requiring enzyme involved in biosynthesis of bacterial lipopolysaccharide. After returning to Japan, he rejoined Sankyo and, together with Masao Kuroda, started his search for a microbial inhibitor of cholesterol biosynthesis.

Discovery of compactin

Endo's premise that inhibition of HMG CoA reductase would lower plasma cholesterol was based on work emanating from the University of Texas in Dallas in the 1960s and was buttressed by Goldstein and Brown's discovery there in 1973 that the monogenic disorder familial hypercholesterolaemia (FH) is characterized by defective regulation of HMG CoA reductase. Using the cultured fibroblast system which they had devised, they and Endo and his colleagues showed compactin to be a potent inhibitor of cholesterol synthesis in vitro in cells from both normal subjects and patients with homozygous FH.[3,4] Initial in vivo studies in mice and rats were, disappointingly, negative,[5] but Endo persevered and showed that compactin lowered serum cholesterol levels in dogs and monkeys.[6,7]

Interestingly enough, compactin had been isolated from a different mould by scientists at Beecham Laboratories in Britain at about the same time as Endo's discovery in Japan.[8] However, they did not get around to investigating its effects on cholesterol synthesis until 1980 and lost interest in the compound when it failed to lower serum cholesterol in mice and rats,[9] despite evidence from John Betteridge and his colleagues at Bart's that it inhibited cholesterol synthesis in human tissue.[10] Without doubt this was a missed opportunity.

The first clinical studies with compactin were carried out in Osaka by Yamamoto and Sudo in collaboration with Endo.[11] They showed that compactin in doses of 50–150 mg/day reduced serum cholesterol by 27% on average in patients with heterozygous FH or combined hyperlipidaemia, most of the decrease being in low-density lipoprotein (LDL) cholesterol. Higher doses were needed to lower cholesterol significantly in FH homozygotes, one of whom developed myopathy, which resolved when the dose of compactin was reduced from 500 to 200 mg daily. However, at that stage, Sankyo suddenly suspended their clinical trial programme, reputedly because of the perceived carcinogenicity of high doses of compactin in dogs. As a consequence, it was never licensed for use in man.

Lovastatin and Merck

Endo left Sankyo in 1978 for an Associate Professorship in the School of Agriculture of Tokyo Noko University, where he continued his studies of fungal inhibitors of cholesterol synthesis. He had collaborated with the US drug company Merck several years previously by providing samples of compactin. The head of research at Merck, Roy Vagelos, had a long-standing interest in HMG CoA reductase, and, like Endo and before him Popjak, he realized the therapeutic potential of inhibiting this enzyme. In 1980, his close colleague Alberts and others at Merck discovered a second HMG CoA reductase inhibitor, which they isolated from *Aspergillus terreus*.[12] This was initially called 'mevinolin' but was later renamed 'lovastatin'. Endo isolated the same compound simultaneously but independently from a different mould, naming it 'monocolin K'.[13] He went on to discover several other HMG CoA reductase inhibitors over the next few years, became a full professor in 1986, and retired from the university in 1997.

Merck proceeded with the clinical development of lovastatin, but the suspension of all clinical studies on compactin by Sankyo put them in a quandary, especially since Sankyo would not disclose the reason. After much deliberation, as described in detail by Steinberg,[8] Merck followed suit and stopped all clinical work while they undertook additional safety studies in animals. The results were sufficiently reassuring for them to resume clinical trials with lovastatin in 1983. These trials were meticulously planned and supervised by Jonathan Tobert, an expatriate clinical pharmacologist from Britain. Four years later, lovastatin became the first HMG CoA reductase inhibitor to be licensed by the US Food and Drug Administration (FDA),[14] an event which was recorded on the cover of *Reader's Digest* (Figure 7.1).

During the interim, Tobert arranged for the compound to be made available to treat patients with refractory FH on a named-patient basis, and I and my Hammersmith colleagues gratefully took advantage of this facility from 1983 onwards, with encouraging results.[15] Using radiolabelled LDL, we and others showed that by inhibiting HMG CoA reductase, lovastatin stimulated receptor-mediated LDL catabolism in vivo, thereby compensating for the inherent deficiency of LDL receptors in FH patients. The ability to treat these severely hypercholesterolaemic patients effectively and safely with such a well tolerated compound represented a major therapeutic advance, especially since its LDL-lowering effect of over 30% was additive to that of existing therapies such as cholestyramine, partial ileal bypass and plasma

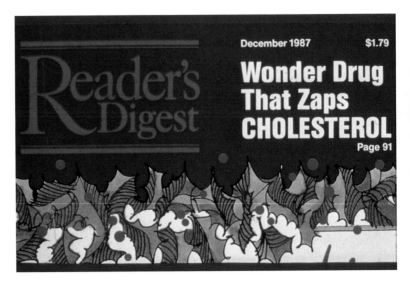

exchange. However, like Yamamoto et al, we found that FH homozygotes were less responsive than heterozygotes.

Because of patent constraints, lovastatin was never licensed in Britain, but Merck maintained supplies for compassionate use until 1989, when its successor simvastatin was licensed in this country. Simvastatin is a semisynthetic derivative of lovastatin, differing only in having an additional methyl group, which prolongs its duration of action. As will become clear later, it was this compound more than any other which helped to vindicate the lipid hypothesis.

Other statins

Other statins soon followed, including pravastatin in 1991, which was derived from compactin and developed by Sankyo; fluvastatin in 1994, which was the first synthetic HMG CoA reductase inhibitor; atorvastatin in 1997; and rosuvastatin in 2003, the latest and most potent of these compounds to be licensed and capable of reducing LDL by over 50%. Cerivastatin was licensed in 1998 but then withdrawn by its manufacturers on account of its myotoxicity, as described later. The latter is the only serious side-effect of statins, but, cerivastatin apart, it is rare, with an incidence of under 0.1%.[14] The myositis is reversible when the statin is stopped, but if not diagnosed it can lead to rhabdomyolysis, renal failure and sometimes death.

The discovery of compactin by Endo has resulted in huge profits for the pharmaceutical industry, but it was not always plain sailing. In addition to early concerns over the suspected toxicity of compactin and the withdrawal of cerivastatin for safety reasons, atorvastatin was nearly scrapped by its developer, Parke-Davis, on economic grounds. It is said that Roger Newton, who was deeply involved in its development, literally went down on his knees before the board to plead for its continuation. The directors relented and it became the best-selling drug in the world.

A first in anti-atherosclerosis therapy

Almost a century and a half ago, Mark Twain summed up the essence of research in these words:

> Discovery! To know that you are walking where none others have walked; that you are beholding what human eye has not seen before ... to discover a great thought, an intellectual nugget, right under the dust of a field that many a brain-plough has gone over before.... To be the first – that is the idea.[16]

Akira Endo's discovery of the hypocholesterolaemic properties of *Penicillium citrinum* over 30 years ago was undoubtedly a first in the prevention and cure of atherosclerotic cardiovascular disease, just as Alexander Fleming's discovery half a century earlier of the antibiotic properties of *Penicillium notatum* revolutionized the treatment of bacterial infections. Many consider that Endo is just as deserving of the Nobel Prize as was Fleming, but, unlike the latter, he has not yet received it. Fittingly, however, he was awarded the Japan Prize in 2006, thereby disproving the adage that a prophet is without honour in his own country.

References

1. Endo A, Kuroda M, Tsujita Y. ML-236A, ML-236B, and ML-236C, new inhibitors of cholesterogenesis produced by *Penicillium citrinum*. *J Antibiot* 1976; **29**: 1346–8.
2. Endo A, Kuroda M, Tanzawa K. Competitive inhibition of 3-hydroxy-3-methylglutaryl coenzyme A reductase by ML-236A and ML-236B fungal metabolites, having hypocholesterolemic activity. *FEBS Lett* 1976; **72**: 323–6.
3. Kaneko I, Hazama-Shimada Y, Endo A. Inhibitory effects on lipid metabolism in cultured cells of ML-236B, a potent inhibitor of 3-hydroxy-3-methylgutaryl-coenzyme-A reductase. *Eur J Biochem* 1978; **87**: 313–21.
4. Brown MS, Faust JR, Goldstein JL, et al. Induction of 3-hydroxy-3-methylglutaryl coenzyme A reductase activity in human fibroblasts

incubated with compactin (ML-236B), a competitive inhibitor of the reductase. *J Biol Chem* 1978; **253**: 1121–8.

5. Endo A, Tsujita Y, Kuroda M, Tanzawa K. Effects of ML-236B on cholesterol metabolism in mice and rats: lack of hypocholesterolemic activity in normal animals. *Biochim Biophys Acta* 1979; **575**: 266–76.

6. Tsujita Y, Kuroda M, Tanzawa K, et al. Hypolipidemic effects in dogs of ML-236B, a competitive inhibitor of 3-hydroxy-3-methyl-glutaryl coenzyme A reductase. *Atherosclerosis* 1979; **32**: 307–13.

7. Kuroda M, Tsujita Y, Tanzawa K, Endo A. Hypolipidemic effects in monkeys of ML-236B, a competitive inhibitor of 3-hydroxy-3-methylglutaryl coenzyme A reductase. *Lipids* 1979; **14**: 585–9.

8. Steinberg D. An interpretative history of the cholesterol controversy. V. The discovery of the statins and the end of the controversy. *J Lipid Res* 2006; **47**: 1339–51.

9. Fears R, Richards DH, Ferres H. The effect of compactin, a potent inhibitor of 3-hydroxy-3-methylglutaryl coenzyme-A reductase activity, on cholesterogenesis and serum cholesterol levels in rats and chicks. *Atherosclerosis* 1980; **35**: 439–49.

10. Betteridge DJ, Krone W, Reckless JPD, Galton DJ. Compactin inhibits cholesterol synthesis in lymphocytes and intestinal mucosa from patients with familial hypercholesterolaemia. *Lancet* 1978; **2**: 1342–3.

11. Yamamoto A, Sudo H, Endo A. Therapeutic effects of ML-236B in primary hypercholesterolemia. *Atherosclerosis* 1980; **35**: 259–66.

12. Alberts AW, Chen J, Kuron G, et al. Mevinolin: a highly potent competitive inhibitor of hydroxymethylglutaryl-coenzyme A reductase and a cholesterol-lowering agent. *Proc Natl Acad Sci U S A* 1980; **77**: 3957–61.

13. Endo A, Monacolin K. A new hypocholesterolemic agent produced by a *Monascus* species. *J Antibiot* 1979; **32**: 852–4.

14. Tobert JA. Lovastatin and beyond: the history of the HMG-CoA reductase inhibitors. *Nat Rev Drug Discov* 2003; **2**: 517–26.

15. Thompson GR, Ford J, Jenkinson M, Trayner I. Efficacy of mevinolin as adjuvant therapy for refractory familial hypercholesterolaemia. *Q J Med* 1986; **60**: 803–11.

16. Mark Twain. *The Innocents Abroad*. London: John Camden Hotten, 1869.

CHAPTER 8

Low cholesterol, murder and suicide

Misinterpretation of an association shown to be due to confounding

Chapter summary

- 'Consensus or nonsensus'
- Cholesterol reduction and non-cardio-vascular mortality
- Public and professional anxiety
- Fuelling the controversy

The contrast between the persistently high death rate from coronary heart disease in England and Wales during the 1970s and rapidly falling rates in the USA and Australia led epidemiologists such as Geoffrey Rose to advocate the mass strategy or population approach to coronary prevention in Britain. This was based on the premise that, in overall terms, many more deaths occur in the large proportion of the population at low risk than in the much smaller proportion at high risk.[1] In contrast, Oliver, a clinician, supported the high-risk strategy, taking the view that the negative outcome of multifactorial risk factor intervention trials meant that the population approach would not work in practice, and discounting claims that the reduction in coronary mortality in the USA might have been due to lifestyle changes.[2] This view was reflected in 1987 by the recommendations of the British Cardiac Society Working Group on Coronary Prevention, of which he was the convener,[3] whereas the European Atherosclerosis Society and the British Hyperlipidaemia Association both supported a combined high-risk and population approach.[4,5]

'Consensus or nonsensus'

Two years earlier, the US National Institutes of Health (NIH) had held a consensus conference on lowering blood cholesterol to prevent heart disease, under the chairmanship of Dan Steinberg.[6] This concluded that elevated blood cholesterol levels are a major cause of coronary disease and that lowering them would reduce the risk of heart attacks. It went on to recommend cholesterol screening and the treatment with diet or drugs of those found to have a raised value, as well as the adoption of dietary measures aimed at lowering the cholesterol level of the entire US population.

The findings of the consensus conference were criticized by Oliver[7] ('consensus or nonsensus') on the grounds that the outcome had been predetermined by the choice of experts invited to participate, although the various alternatives he proposed all seemed liable to the same source of bias. He later switched his line of attack on American efforts to prevent coronary heart disease by invoking safety concerns, pointing out that while lowering serum cholesterol reduced coronary mortality it failed to decrease total mortality, perhaps by increasing non-cardiovascular causes of death.[8] He went on to suggest that the presence of low cholesterol in patients with cancer was not necessarily a post-hoc phenomenon and that therapeutic lowering of serum cholesterol might sometimes cause cancer, possibly by altering the cholesterol content of cell membranes. The concept that lowering serum cholesterol might be carcinogenic was not new but dated from the Los Angeles Veterans Administration trial conducted 20 years previously, where an increased risk of developing cancer was observed in men on a diet high in polyunsaturated fat. It so happened that the expression of these safety concerns was the prelude to a major escalation in hostilities on the cholesterol front.

Cholesterol reduction and non-cardiovascular mortality

In 1990, Muldoon and two of his colleagues at the University of Pittsburgh, a psychologist and a psychiatrist, published in the *British Medical Journal* a meta-analysis of six primary prevention trials of cholesterol reduction, two using diet and four using drugs.[9] Coronary mortality was shown to be significantly reduced by drug treatment, but total mortality was unchanged. This reflected the fact that there was a significant increase in deaths from accidents, suicide and violence in those on treatment, although there was no correlation between cholesterol reduction and deaths from cancer. The authors were unable to provide a plausible explanation as to why lowering serum cholesterol should predispose to violent deaths, but they considered the possibility that it did so by altering neuronal function. They subsequently suggested that cholesterol-lowering manoeuvres might reduce brain serotoninergic activity and thereby promote suicidal behaviour and aggressive tendencies.[10]

One of the studies analysed in Muldoon's original meta-analysis was the Minnesota Coronary Survey, during which inmates of six mental hospitals who had been on a lipid-lowering diet for just over a year had a significant excess of accidental deaths compared with inmates not on the diet. The causes of death included fractures, drug reactions, burns, foreign bodies, tooth extractions, freezing, heatstroke, drowning and suicide. It is hard to conceive of a unifying causal mechanism which could account for such a bizarre and disparate series of fatal events.[11]

Evidence from other sources did not support the findings of Muldoon et al. In the Whitehall Study, almost 18 000 men were followed up for 20 years, during which 90 died from accidents, violence or suicide. No significant association was seen between these deaths and serum cholesterol at entry to the study.[12] A large Swedish study did find a negative correlation between serum cholesterol at entry and suicide within the next 7 years, but not during the remainder of the 20 years of follow-up, and the increased risk of suicide was seen only in men, not in women.[13] A similar study in Finland showed no association between serum cholesterol and violent deaths or suicides during 10–15 years of follow-up but found these deaths to be more prevalent among smokers and drinkers.[14] These findings may have reassured some, but not Michael Oliver, who continued to sound the alarm in editorials with titles such as 'Might treatment of hypercholesterolaemia increase non-cardiac mortality?' and 'Is cholesterol reduction always safe?'[15,16]

Anxieties over this issue were suddenly brought to public attention in 1992 with the publication of an article by George Davey Smith and Juha Pekkanen titled 'Should there be a moratorium on the use of cholesterol lowering drugs?'[17] This was at a time when the development of statins was proceeding at a rapid pace and clinical trials with lovastatin, simvastatin and pravastatin were under way. Davey Smith and Pekkanen had conducted a meta-analysis similar to but larger than Muldoon's, including additional data from diet and drug trials. They confirmed that coronary mortality was reduced by lowering cholesterol in both types of trial and that total mortality was unchanged. However, they also reported a highly significant increase in non-coronary mortality, reflecting an amalgam of cancer, injury and other non-cardiovascular causes of death in the intervention groups of the drug trials, but not the diet trials. This led them to question whether the general use of cholesterol-lowering drugs was justified and to propose that the prescription of these agents should be restricted to patients with familial hyperlipidaemia until the results of the statin trials became known, still some years hence.

Public and professional anxiety

The publication of this paper in the *British Medical Journal* resulted in an immediate plethora of hyperbolical headlines in the newspapers, ranging from 'Heart pills may kill you' to 'Murders linked to low-fat drugs', causing panic among patients who were on cholesterol-lowering medication and disquiet to their doctors (Figure 8.1). Public and professional anxiety regarding the safety of these compounds persisted until 1994, when Malcolm Law and his colleagues conducted an exhaustively thorough, systematic review of 40 published studies.[18] Apart from an unexplained increase in the risk of fatal haemorrhagic stroke in hypertensive subjects, they found no evidence that lowering or having low cholesterol increased mortality from any cause. They attributed the associations between low serum cholesterol and both cancer and suicide to confounding, inasmuch as low serum cholesterol is often a consequence of cancer or of dietary neglect, the latter being a common finding in depressed subjects with suicidal tendencies. An accompanying editorial in the *British Medical Journal* damned these conclusions with faint praise by its subtitle: 'Lowering population cholesterol concentrations probably isn't harmful'.[19]

Figure 8.1 *Newspaper headlines in 1992 following the publication of a paper by Davey Smith and Pekkanen in the* British Medical Journal

For conveying the impression that the excess mortality in a number of the drug trials was spurious, Law et al were criticized by Oliver and his colleagues, who emphasized that the increased mortality of subjects on clofibrate in the WHO trial was genuine,[20] whereas Davey Smith and Egger took issue with them

THE DAILY TELEGRAPH 15TH FEBRUARY 1992	**Cholesterol drugs 'risk to patients'**
THE TIMES 14TH FEBRUARY 1992	Heart pills can increase risk of death
THE STAR 14TH FEBRUARY 1992	*HEART PILLS MAY KILL YOU*
THE GUARDIAN 14TH FEBRUARY 1992	**Murders linked to low-fat drugs**

on their use of statistics.[21] Muldoon, too, was initially reluctant to accept that cholesterol-lowering measures were safe, but he and his colleagues later acknowledged that 'currently available evidence does not indicate that non-cholesterol illness mortality is increased significantly by cholesterol lowering treatments'.[22] Despite the criticisms, Law's analysis did a great deal to reassure those responsible for prescribing lipid-lowering drugs at a time when the latter were under intense scrutiny and the safety of statins was still an unknown quantity.

Fuelling the controversy

Public unease about cholesterol continued, however, fuelled by individuals within the medical profession and news media alike. This was exemplified by an article in the *Sunday Express* in 1990 with the pejorative title 'Exploding the cholesterol myth'.[23] The medical editor who wrote the article suggested that 'raised cholesterol might be a symptom, rather than a cause, of a state in which heart disease became likely.... Raised levels of circulating cholesterol should be seen as a reflection of the over-taxed body's attempts to cope with these demands.' The article went on to point out that lowering cholesterol might be harmful and concluded, 'because of the hazards of long-term treatment, the wise patient will make every effort to come off the drugs as soon as possible'. The likely source of this pseudoscientific nonsense is revealed in the following excerpts from a letter written that year by a consultant cardiologist at a London teaching hospital to one of his patients:

> Dear Mr C
>
> This is just a letter to confirm my opinion that you live with high levels of adrenergic drive by habit, sufficiently high as to carry you over the top of the curve into catabolic territory where the cholesterol level naturally climbs....
>
> If you learned to live at the peak instead of on the downslope of the curve I would expect your cholesterol levels to regress from their excursions towards a mean. As far as I know, this mean may be within the normal range of values.

One must assume that the journalist picked up this gobbledegook from the cardiologist rather than vice versa. Unfortunately, some believed what they read, including a patient who had undergone coronary bypass surgery and whose hypercholesterolaemia was being treated at a Northampton hospital. The consultant in charge wrote to the newspaper's editor, complaining that his patient had discontinued all cholesterol-lowering medication after reading the article in question and was now untreated. The likelihood is that other patients reacted in a similar manner, with potentially serious consequences. These anecdotes illustrate that the cholesterol controversy was by no means over at the start of the 1990s and that it continued to influence the actions of doctors and patients alike.

References

1. Rose G. Strategy of prevention: lessons from cardiovascular disease. *Br Med J* 1981; **282**: 1847–51.
2. Oliver MF. Should we not forget about mass control of coronary risk factors? *Lancet* 1983; **2**: 37–8.
3. British Cardiac Society Working Group on Coronary Prevention. Conclusions and recommendations. *Br Heart J* 1987; **57**: 188–9.
4. Study Group, European Atherosclerosis Society. Strategies for the prevention of coronary heart disease: a policy statement of the European Atherosclerosis Society. *Eur Heart J* 1987; **8**: 77–88.
5. Shepherd J, Betteridge DJ, Durrington P, et al. Strategies for reducing coronary heart disease and desirable limits for blood lipid concentrations: guidelines of the British Hyperlipidaemia Association. *Br Med J* 1987; **295**: 1245–6.
6. Consensus conference. Lowering blood cholesterol to prevent heart disease. *JAMA* 1985; **253**: 2080–6.
7. Oliver MF. Consensus or nonsensus – conferences on coronary heart disease. *Lancet* 1985; **1**: 1087–9.
8. Oliver MF. Reducing cholesterol does not reduce mortality. *J Am Coll Cardiol* 1988; **12**: 814–17.
9. Muldoon MF, Manuck SB, Matthews KA. Lowering cholesterol concentrations and mortality: a quantitative review of primary prevention trials. *Br Med J* 1990; **301**: 309–14.
10. Muldoon MF, Rossouw JE, Manuck CB, et al. Low or lowered cholesterol and risk of death from suicide and trauma. *Metabolism* 1993; **42**(Suppl 1): 45–56.
11. Thompson GR. Cholesterol lowering and non-cardiac mortality [Letter]. *Lancet* 1991; **2**: 126.
12. Davey Smith G, Shipley MJ, et al. Lowering cholesterol concentrations and mortality [Letter]. *Br Med J* 1990; **301**: 552.
13. Lindberg G, Rastam L, Gullberg B, Eklund GA. Low serum cholesterol concentrations and short term mortality from injuries in men and women. *Br Med J* 1992; **305**: 277–9.
14. Vartiainen E, Puska P, Pekkanen J, et al. Serum cholesterol concentration and mortality from accidents, suicide, and other violent causes. *Br Med J* 1994; **309**: 445–7.
15. Oliver MF. Might treatment of hypercholesterolaemia increase non-cardiac mortality? *Lancet* 1991; **337**: 1529–31.
16. Oliver MF. Is cholesterol reduction always safe? *Eur J Clin Invest* 1992; **22**: 441–2.

17. Davey Smith G, Pekkanen J. Should there be a moratorium on the use of cholesterol lowering drugs? *Br Med J* 1992; **304**: 431–4.
18. Law MR, Thompson SG, Wald NJ. Assessing possible hazards of reducing serum cholesterol. *Br Med J* 1994; **308**: 373–9.
19. Marmot M. The cholesterol papers. *Br Med J* 1994; **308**: 351–2.
20. Heady JA, Morris JN, Oliver MF. Ischaemic heart disease and cholesterol. There's more to heart disease than cholesterol. … and mislead on adverse effects [Letter]. *Br Med J* 1994; **308**: 1040.
21. Davey Smith G, Egger M. Commentary: statistical problems. *Br Med J* 1994; **308**: 1025–7.
22. Muldoon MF, Manuck SB, Mendelsohn AB, et al. Cholesterol reduction and non-illness mortality: meta-analysis of randomised clinical trials. *Br Med J* 2001; **322**: 11–15.
23. Hodgkinson N. Exploding the cholesterol myth. *Sunday Express*, 4 February 1990.

CHAPTER 9

The statin trials

The unequivocal outcome of 4S, WOSCOPS and HPS proves the lipid hypothesis

Chapter summary

- Regression trials
- Plaque composition and clinical events
- Impact of 4S
- WOSCOPS
- The Heart Protection Study
- The final proof

D espite the efforts of epidemiologists such as Morris, Rose and Shaper, many cardiologists remained unconvinced that lowering cholesterol by diet or drugs would provide an effective, let alone safe, means of treating and preventing coronary heart disease. However, some did consider that cholesterol might play a causal role in atherosclerosis and decided to test this hypothesis by undertaking so-called regression trials, in which the impact of cholesterol-lowering measures on hyperlipidaemic patients with coronary artery disease was assessed angiographically. The main instigator of these trials was the late David Blankenhorn from Los Angeles, generally regarded as the founding father of studies of atherosclerosis regression in humans.

Regression trials

The results of a dozen such studies were reported between 1984 and 1994, most of them from the USA.[1] These ranged in size from less than 50 to over 800 subjects and lasted between 1 and 10 years. Most involved a randomized comparison of diet and diet combined with lipid-lowering drugs. Alternative forms of treatment included partial ileal bypass, exercise and anti-stress measures. In the earlier trials, bile acid sequestrants, such as cholestyramine and colestipol, were given alone or in combination with either nicotinic acid or lovastatin. In later trials, lovastatin or simvastatin was given as monotherapy. In the earlier trials, angiographic changes were assessed visually, whereas later ones used computer-assisted quantitative coronary angiography (QCA).

Baseline levels of serum total and low-density lipoprotein (LDL) cholesterol varied considerably between the 12 trials, with overall means of 6.3 and 4.4 mmol/l, respectively. During the trials, LDL cholesterol was 31% lower and high-density lipoprotein (HDL) cholesterol 5% higher in the intervention groups than in the controls. Angiographic criteria varied, but all patients were categorized according to whether their coronary lesions showed progression, regression, mixed response or no change. Of the more than 2500 patients involved, 44% of the controls were classified as progressors and 9% as regressors, compared with 29% and 18%, respectively, of those on treatment. Hence lipid-lowering treatment reduced the chances of progression by one-third and increased the chances of regression twofold. In those trials which used QCA, the minimum diameter of lesions narrowed less on treatment than in controls (by –0.02 versus –0.09 mm) and percentage diameter stenosis increased less (by 0.7% versus 2.6%). Therefore, lipid-lowering therapy reduced progression rather than induced regression.

Plaque composition and clinical events

Although not powered to detect changes in clinical end points, three trials[2-4] did show a significant reduction in cardiovascular events and in the need for revascularization procedures. Greg Brown and colleagues in Seattle examined the relation between clinical events and plaque size in one of these trials, the Familial Atherosclerosis Treatment Study (FATS),[3] and concluded that mildly to moderately stenosed lesions were usually the culprits and were more responsive to lipid-lowering therapy than were severe (>70% stenosed) lesions.[5]

As was shown by the late Michael Davies and his colleagues in London, high-grade stenotic lesions contain large amounts of collagen and calcium but relatively little lipid, whereas the propensity of plaques to undergo fissuring and thrombosis, and thereby precipitate a clinical event, was determined by the amount of extracellular lipid in the core of the plaque.[6] Thus, a reduction in the amount of lipid in moderately stenotic lesions resulting in only a modest decrease in plaque size should be accompanied by an increase in plaque stability and a reduction in clinical events, as occurred in FATS. In all probability, the relatively slight quantitative changes in vessel lumen in the regression trials were haemodynamically insignificant; nevertheless, they appear to have been an important marker of plaque stabilization.

In September 1992, a joint meeting of the British Atherosclerosis Discussion Group and the European Atherosclerosis

Society was held at Downing College in Cambridge. The topic was 'Regression of atherosclerosis' and the participants included David Blankenhorn, Greg Brown, Michael Davies and Neville Woolf, all of whom had made major contributions in this field. The careful pathological studies of Davies and Woolf were especially important in showing that lesion composition, rather than size, was the main factor in determining clinical events. All were agreed that regression trials such as FATS provided a strong hint that lipid lowering could reduce coronary events, but the question of whether or not this would be accompanied by a reduction in total mortality, the Holy Grail of preventive strategies, was still unresolved. The answer was not long in coming, however, and it came from Scandinavia.

Impact of 4S

In the autumn of 1994, *The Lancet* published the results of the Scandinavian Simvastatin Survival Study (4S), which provided unequivocal evidence that treatment of hypercholesterolaemia in patients with existing coronary heart disease reduced both cardiovascular events and total mortality.[7] In this epic trial, 4444 mostly male patients from Denmark, Finland, Iceland, Norway and Sweden, aged 35–70, with angina or previous myocardial infarction and with serum cholesterol averaging 6.8 mmol/l on diet, were randomized to receive simvastatin or placebo. Simvastatin dosage was initially 20 mg/day but was increased to 40 mg/day as necessary, so as to maintain serum cholesterol in the range 3–5.2 mmol/l. During the study, simvastatin reduced total cholesterol by 25% and LDL cholesterol by 35% and increased HDL cholesterol by 8%.

The median duration of treatment was 5.4 years, after which the trial was stopped because of a highly significant 30% reduction in total mortality. This was entirely due to a 42% reduction in coronary mortality, and there was no increase in non-cardiovascular causes of death, including cancer and trauma. In addition to its effects on coronary disease, simvastatin significantly reduced the occurrence of cerebrovascular events. The mean level of LDL cholesterol with simvastatin in 4S was 3.2 mmol/l, similar to the 3 mmol/l seen in the regression trials. Taken together, these findings showed that a 30–35% reduction in LDL cholesterol resulted in decreased progression of coronary atheromatous lesions and fewer clinical events; the 4S authors estimated that simvastatin had prevented 4 out of every 9 deaths that otherwise would have occurred.

The publication of the 4S results had an immediate impact on medical practice (Figure 9.1). Even Michael Oliver was

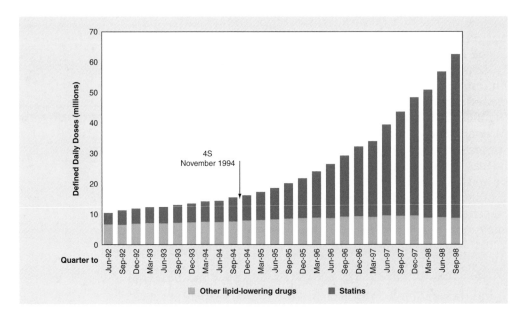

Figure 9.1 *Exponential increase in prescribing of statins in England following publication of the results of 4S in 1994 (reproduced with permission from Ferguson J,* British Journal of Cardiolology *1999;6:459–65)*

impressed, and he was co-author of an article in the *British Medical Journal* entitled 'Lower patients' cholesterol now'.[8] However, this included a caveat that the increase in non-cardiovascular mortality seen in primary prevention trials of cholesterol lowering was still an issue to be resolved. An answer would soon be forthcoming, as he would have known in his role as Chairman of the Data and Safety Monitoring Committee of the West of Scotland Coronary Prevention Study (WOSCOPS).[9]

WOSCOPS

According to Chris Packard,[10] WOSCOPS was conceived by James (Jim) Shepherd at the Glasgow Royal Infirmary in 1988 during a visit there by James Hill, a senior director of Squibb, the licensee in Britain of pravastatin. At that meeting, the local cardiologists voted for a secondary prevention trial with pravastatin, but Squibb had already decided to do one elsewhere. Jim Shepherd, however, suggested that a primary prevention trial was needed, an idea which appealed to Squibb. They decided to back his proposal, and as a result WOSCOPS became the first primary prevention trial to use a statin. This initially involved screening more than 80 000 men in the West of Scotland, of whom 6595 were selected on the basis of being asymptomatic, aged 45–64 and having serum total cholesterol over 6.5 mmol/l and LDL cholesterol of 4.5–6 mmol/l. They were then randomized to receive pravastatin 40 mg/day or placebo for an average duration of just under 5 years.

The results were published in 1995, exactly a year after the publication of 4S. Pravastatin decreased serum total and LDL cholesterol by 20% and 26%, respectively, and raised HDL cholesterol by 5%. These changes were associated with a highly significant 31% reduction in non-fatal myocardial infarcts plus coronary deaths. Although the 22% reduction in total mortality just failed to achieve statistical significance, there was no increase in non-cardiovascular causes of death in pravastatin-treated subjects.

Oliver's commentary on this occasion was entitled 'Statins prevent coronary heart disease',[11] but he remained reluctant to draw any conclusions about non-cardiac mortality, opting to wait for the results of the Heart Protection Study, still several years hence. However, he relented before then at a meeting held in Stockholm in 1996 to celebrate the tenth anniversary of the award of the Nobel Prize to Goldstein and Brown. It was there that he finally completed his U-turn, which he justified by citing Maynard Keynes: 'When the facts change, I change my mind. What do you do?'

The Heart Protection Study

Several other statin trials were published between 1995 and 1998, but the largest of them was not completed until the start of the new millennium. This was the Medical Research Council/British Heart Foundation Heart Protection Study (HPS),[12] which was designed and conducted by the Oxford-based Clinical Trials Service Unit, with Rory Collins as the principal investigator. This trial examined the effects on mortality and morbidity of cholesterol-lowering therapy in more than 20000 subjects with, or at high risk of, cardiovascular disease in the UK. Men and women aged 40–80 with serum total cholesterol over 3.5 mmol/l were randomized to receive either simvastatin 40 mg daily or anti-oxidant vitamins, the two combined, or placebo.

The results showed an incidence of major coronary events in those on placebo of 11.8% over 5 years, confirming that they were a high-risk group. Subjects allocated to simvastatin had a mean reduction in LDL cholesterol of 1 mmol/l, with decreases in total and cardiovascular mortality of 12% and 17% and decreases in coronary events and strokes of 26% and 27%, respectively. Benefit from simvastatin occurred irrespective of the level of LDL cholesterol at entry to the study, and was not influenced by age, gender or clinical status, and there was no increase in non-cardio-vascular mortality. One-third of the patients in the HPS had a baseline LDL cholesterol under 3 mmol/l, an important finding suggesting that high-risk individuals benefit from LDL lowering even if their LDL cholesterol is 'normal'.

The final proof

The final dotting of '*i*'s and crossing of '*t*'s that marked the end of the controversy over the lipid hypothesis came when data from over 90 000 individuals who participated in 14 statin trials in 1994–2004 were meta-analysed by the Cholesterol Treatment Trialists' Collaboration.[13] The results showed decreases of 12% and 19% in total and coronary mortality, respectively, for each 1 mmol/l reduction in LDL cholesterol, similar to what was found in the HPS. Overall, the risk of a major vascular event, including stroke, was reduced by one-fifth. No significant changes in non-cardiovascular mortality occurred over the 5-year duration of these trials, and one feels that even McMichael and Mitchell would have been impressed by these data, while Oliver preserved an eloquent silence.

Which brings us back to 1953, when Oliver and Boyd first presented their findings showing an association between raised cholesterol and coronary disease in British men. That was the year that Pollak published a paper describing for the first time the cholesterol-lowering properties of plant sterols, which he concluded with this forecast: 'Some day, the question as to the value of prophylactic or therapeutic reduction of blood cholesterol will be answered.'[14] He was right – more than 50 years later it has been.

References

1. Thompson GR. Angiographic trials of lipid-lowering therapy: end of an era? *Br Heart J* 1995; **74**: 343–7.
2. Buchwald H, Varco RL, Matts JP, et al. Effect of partial ileal bypass surgery on mortality and morbidity from coronary heart disease in patients with hypercholesterolemia. *N Engl J Med* 1990; **323**: 946–55.
3. Brown G, Alberts JJ, Fisher LD. Regression of coronary artery disease as a result of intensive lipid-lowering therapy in men with high levels of apolipoprotein B. *N Engl J Med* 1990; **323**: 1289–98.
4. Watts GF, Lewis B, Brunt JNH, et al. Effects on coronary artery disease of lipid-lowering diet, or diet plus cholestyramine in the St. Thomas' Atherosclerosis Regression Study (STARS). *Lancet* 1992; **339**: 563–9.
5. Brown BG, Zhao X-Q, Sacco DE, Albers JJ. Atherosclerosis regression, plaque disruption, and cardiovascular events. A rationale for lipid

lowering in coronary artery disease. *Annu Rev Med* 1993; **44**: 365–76.

6. Davies MJ, Krikler DM, Katz D. Atherosclerosis: inhibition or regression as therapeutic possibilities. *Br Heart J* 1991; **65**: 302–10.

7. Scandinavian Simvastatin Survival Study Group. Randomised trial of cholesterol lowering in 4444 patients with coronary heart disease: the Scandinavian Simvastatin Survival Study (4S). *Lancet* 1994; **344**: 1383–9.

8. Oliver M, Poole-Wilson P, Shepherd J, Tikkanen M. Lower patients' cholesterol now. *Br Med J* 1995; **310**: 1280–1.

9. Shepherd J, Cobbe SM, Ford I, et al. Prevention of coronary heart disease with pravastatin in men with hypercholesterolemia. West of Scotland Coronary Prevention Study Group. *N Engl J Med* 1995; **333**: 1301–7.

10. Packard C. Cholesterol, atherosclerosis and coronary disease in the UK, 1950–2000. In Reynolds LA, Tansey EM, eds. *Wellcome Witnesses to Twentieth Century Medicine* 2006; **27**: 77.

11. Oliver MF. Statins prevent coronary heart disease. *Lancet* 1995; **346**: 1378–9.

12. Heart Protection Study Collaborative Group. MRC/BHF heart protection study of cholesterol lowering with simvastatin in 20536 high-risk individuals: a randomised placebo-controlled trial. *Lancet* 2002; **360**: 7–22.

13. Baigent C, Keech A, Kearney PM, et al. Efficacy and safety of cholesterol-lowering treatment: prospective meta-analysis of data from 90,056 participants in 14 randomised trials of statins. *Lancet* 2005; **366**: 1267–78.

14. Pollak OJ. Reduction of blood cholesterol in man. *Circulation* 1953; **7**: 702–6.

CHAPTER 10

Demise of a statin
Muscle toxicity of cerivastatin leads to its withdrawal

Chapter summary

- Cerivastatin is launched
- Cerivastatin is withdrawn
- Myotoxicity of other statins
- Fibrate–statin interaction
- Mechanism of statin-induced myotoxicity
- Roles of Bayer and the FDA

At the start of 1997, an 'International Top Opinion Leaders Seminar on the Management and Treatment of Dyslipidaemia' took place in the resort of Indian Wells, near Palm Springs, California. The Saturday afternoon session dealt with general topics, but the *raison d'être* of the meeting became apparent the following morning when the sponsor, Bayer, revealed details of its new hydroxymethylglutaryl co-enzyme A (HMG CoA) reductase inhibitor, cerivastatin. Clinical trial data showed that doses of 0.2–0.4 mg daily decreased low-density lipoprotein (LDL) cholesterol by 25–35%, appreciably less than that achieved by a recently licensed competitor, atorvastatin. However, the expectation was that increasing the dose of cerivastatin to 0.8 mg daily would narrow the gap in efficacy without compromising safety, given that this dose was only one-hundredth that of the highest dose of atorvastatin.

In June of that year, the use of cerivastatin 0.2 and 0.3 mg daily was approved in the USA, and in October Bayer held a second Opinion Leaders Seminar, this time in New York. During the meeting, results were presented from a study of hyper-cholesterolaemic patients given cerivastatin 0.8 mg daily for 1 month, which decreased their LDL cholesterol on average by 43%. However, one of the 28 patients had an eightfold increase in serum creatine phosphokinase (CK) levels, which was suggestive of myositis. The latter was known to be a rare but potentially dangerous side-effect of statins, with a rate of occurrence of 0.1–0.2% in clinical trials. In retrospect, the fact that even one, i.e. over 3%, of the patients on cerivastatin 0.8 mg/day developed a raised CK level should have rung warning bells, especially when it became apparent that the toxicologists at Bayer were reluctant to test higher doses. However, the feeling at the time was that they were being overcautious, and in an editorial the following year I suggested that the low dose and dual pathways of metabolism of cerivastatin implied that it had a lesser propensity for drug interactions than other statins, and hence a lower likelihood of myotoxicity.[1] Subsequent events proved that this plausible concept was fallacious.

Cerivastatin is launched

In February 1998, cerivastatin was launched under the trade names Baycol in the USA and Lipobay in Britain and Europe. Just over a year later, the first case of myositis leading to rhabdomyolysis in a patient on cerivastatin was published.[2] This individual was also taking the fibrate gemfibrozil; despite developing renal failure, the patient eventually recovered. It had previously been shown that the chances of developing myositis on lovastatin were increased 20–30-fold by concomitant administration of gemfibrozil,[3] and the authors of the cerivastatin report therefore questioned whether the dual cytochrome P450 pathways (CYP3A4 and CYP2C8), by which this drug was metabolized by the liver, provided any protection against drug interaction. This argument was rebutted by others,[4] who proposed that it was the interaction between cerivastatin and gemfibrozil at the level of the muscle cell that explained the enhanced myotoxicity of these drugs when they were given together.

Bayer's application for a licence to market the 0.8-mg dose of cerivastatin was approved by the US Food and Drug Administration (FDA) in July 2000. One month later, a second case of severe rhabdomyolysis and renal failure was reported in a patient on cerivastatin and gemfibrozil, this time from Turkey and with a fatal outcome.[5] Earlier that year, a group of physicians in Houston, Texas, had switched approximately 3000 patients to cerivastatin from other statins in order to reduce costs. During the following 9 months, they documented six cases of rhabdomyolysis among patients on cerivastatin 0.4 mg daily, none of whom was on gemfibrozil, but observed no cases in patients taking other statins without gemfibrozil.[6] They suggested that cerivastatin had greater myotoxicity than other statins, even in the absence of gemfibrozil.

Cerivastatin is withdrawn

In August 2001, the FDA announced that it had received reports of 31 deaths from rhabdomyolysis in patients taking cerivastatin, a third of whom were also on gemfibrozil, and confirmed that Bayer was voluntarily withdrawing its drug from the US market. A similar announcement was made by the Medicines Control Agency in Britain, which pointed out that Europe-wide action had already been taken to limit the maximum dose of cerivastatin to 0.4 mg daily and to warn against the concomitant use of gemfibrozil. The subsequent publication of the results of a year-long study indicated that even this dose of cerivastatin was unsafe, with CK elevations over 10 times the upper limit of normal in 1.5% of patients, compared with none in those on pravastatin; nor was it particularly effective, achieving reductions in LDL cholesterol of only 34%.[7]

The commercial consequences of the cerivastatin debacle were serious. Its withdrawal reduced Bayer's annual profits by €600 million in 2001, and the company reportedly faced a fine by the German health authorities for withholding information about its interaction with gemfibrozil, an accusation which Bayer denied.[8] The company also faced a criminal prosecution over this issue in Switzerland and possibly elsewhere, in that, in addition to the deaths in the USA, there were over 20 in other parts of the world.[9] In Texas, a court ordered Bayer to release confidential documents during a lawsuit brought by a patient who developed rhabdomyolysis while on cerivastatin, the contents of which proved embarrassing for the company when they were made public.[10] By 2003, Bayer had paid out over $600 million to settle 1600 claims out of court in the USA and was reputedly in danger of incurring charges in excess of its insurance cover. These were very substantial losses, especially when added to the high cost of developing and marketing the drug.

Myotoxicity of other statins

As might have been expected, the sudden demise of cerivastatin soon focused attention on the safety of other statins. Initial reactions were reassuring – for example, Farmer[11] found no difference between placebo and treatment groups in the frequency of myositis or rhabdomyolysis in over 30 000 subjects who had participated in trials of lovastatin, pravastatin and simvastatin. This impression was reinforced by a series of reports from the Office of Drug Safety of the FDA. The first of these used the FDA's adverse event reporting scheme and a national audit of prescriptions to estimate the frequency of fatal rhabdomyolysis in statin users in the USA.[12] The rate varied from 0 to 0.2 per million prescriptions for lovastatin, pravastatin, simvastatin, atorvastatin and fluvastatin, compared with 3.2 per million prescriptions for cerivastatin, representing a 16–80-fold greater risk for patients on the latter drug. If deaths in those receiving concomitant gemfibrozil were excluded, the rate for cerivastatin was 1.9 per million, still 10–50 times that of mono-therapy with other statins. Analysis of the 19 deaths associated with cerivastatin monotherapy revealed that 12 had occurred in patients taking 0.8 mg/day and 6 in those on 0.4 mg/day, suggesting that rhabdomyolysis was dose related.

In a subsequent publication, the same group examined the FDA database for all cases of rhabdomyolysis reported between 1988, when lovastatin first came on the market, and mid-2001, when cerivastatin was withdrawn[13] (Figure 10.1). Of the 866 reported cases, more than 80% were hospitalized, usually with renal failure, and 80 of them died. Over 50% were on statin monotherapy, half of them on cerivastatin, and the remainder were on combination therapy, mainly cerivastatin plus gemfi-brozil. Most of the cerivastatin cases of rhabdomyolysis were in that category.

Figure 10.1 *Cases of rhabdomyolysis associated with statins reported in the USA between January 1988 and July 2001, showing the increased frequency associated with use of cerivas-tatin (reproduced with permission from Chang et al, Pharmacoepidemi-ology and Drug Safety, 2004;13: 417–26. © John Wiley & Sons Ltd)*

Fibrate-statin interaction

In their third paper, the FDA workers reviewed prescription claims and medical records relating to managed health-care schemes in the USA between 1998 and mid-2001.[14] They iden-tified 24 cases of rhabdomyolysis out of a total of 250 000 patients treated with lipid-lowering drugs, of which 13 were on a statin, 3 on a fibrate (all gemfibrozil) and 8 on a statin plus a fibrate. Monotherapy with a fibrate had a fivefold higher risk than monotherapy with statins other than cerivastatin, which carried a 12-fold higher risk than other statins. Concomitant

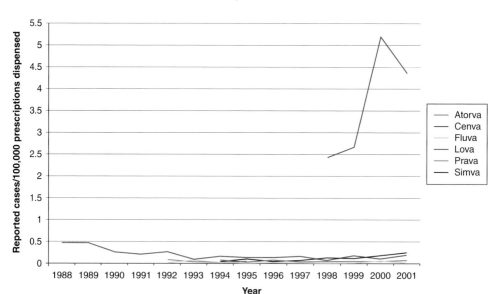

administration of a fibrate increased the risk of rhabdomyolysis in non-cerivastatin statin users 13-fold, and in cerivastatin users almost 200-fold. These data confirmed that cerivastatin was far more myotoxic than other statins and demonstrated that this tendency was greatly enhanced by fibrates. However, only one of the eight cases of rhabdomyolysis on combination therapy was on fenofibrate, suggesting that it might be safer than gemfibrozil in this context.

This issue was addressed by Jones and Davidson,[15] who used a similar approach to the FDA workers[12] to compare the frequency of rhabdomyolysis in patients on statin/fibrate combination therapy. They showed that the rate was 15-fold higher when gemfibrozil rather than fenofibrate was combined with a statin other than cerivastatin and 32-fold higher when combined with cerivastatin. These findings reinforced current opinion that fenofibrate might sometimes be given as an adjunct to a statin, whereas gemfibrozil should never be used for that purpose.

A subsequent meta-analysis by the Cholesterol Treatment Trialists' Collaborators of data from over 90 000 patients was reassuring, inasmuch as it confirmed that most of the statins in current use had a very low risk of rhabdomyolysis.[16] Except, that is, when they were given with other drugs. A review found that almost 60% of cases of statin-induced rhabdomyolysis occurred in patients taking drugs affecting statin metabolism, mainly fibrates, but also including CYP3A4 inhibitors such as cyclosporine, macrolide antibiotics, and azole anti-fungals.[17] These drugs impair the metabolic degradation of lovastatin, simvastatin and atorvastatin, and thereby increase their blood levels. However, the metabolism of cerivastatin is minimally influenced by CYP3A4 inhibitors,[4] a fact that poses further questions regarding the mechanism of statin-induced myotoxicity and how gemfibrozil enhances this effect.

Mechanism of statin-induced myotoxicity

The myotoxic effect of statins is poorly understood. Data obtained in experimental animals and muscle cell preparations in vitro suggest that it probably reflects inhibition of HMG CoA reductase rather than reduced cholesterol synthesis. For example, squalene synthase inhibitors, which block the synthesis of cholesterol, but not HMG CoA reductase, are not myotoxic.[18] This led investigators to examine the effects on muscle of non-cholesterol products of HMG CoA reductase, such as ubiquinone (co-enzyme Q10), synthesis of which is reduced by statins. However, experiments in rats showed no difference in ubiquinone levels in muscles of animals with and without cerivastatin-induced myositis,[19] and a subsequent study attributed the myopathic effect of cerivastatin to inhibition of geranylgeranylation of protein.[20] This process, essential for cell growth, is inhibited by statins, but not by squalene synthase inhibitors. It remains to be shown whether these findings have any clinical relevance.

The mechanism whereby gemfibrozil influences statin metabolism was studied in humans by Backman et al.[21] Pretreatment of healthy volunteers with gemfibrozil followed by a single dose of cerivastatin increased the area under the plasma concentration–time curve (AUC) of cerivastatin fivefold and caused an equivalent decrease in the AUC of its major CYP2C8-dependent metabolite. Studies using human liver cells showed that gemfibrozil not only inhibited the conversion of cerivastatin to its inactive metabolite but also reduced glucuronidation of the parent drug.[22] Interference with these dual excretory pathways would account for the increase in blood levels of cerivastatin when the latter was given together with gemfibrozil, and explain its enhanced myotoxicity.

Roles of Bayer and the FDA

What other lessons can be learned from the cerivastatin saga? At the end of 2004, more than half of an issue of the *Journal of the American Medical Association* was devoted to this question, with particular reference to the roles played by Bayer and the FDA. The revelation of confidential company information provided a unique insight into Bayer's activities, information which became available to Psaty et al[23] in their role as expert witnesses on behalf of patients suing for damages relating to cerivastatin. Important issues which were addressed in their paper and in an accompanying editorial[24] included the post-marketing reporting of adverse drug reactions and the conflict of interest this can engender in drug companies. For example, it was disclosed that Bayer had received reports of six cases of rhabdomyolysis within four months of the launch of cerivastatin, five of which were also on gemfibrozil, but had waited 18 months before sending out a 'Dear Doctor' letter contraindicating the combined use of these drugs.[23] It was also revealed that in July 1999 an unpublished study of cerivastatin 1.6 mg/day documented a raised CK in 12% of recipients, suggesting that the company knew early on that high blood levels of the drug were myotoxic. Despite this, Bayer delayed conducting a pharmacokinetic study of the interaction between cerivastatin and gemfibrozil until April 2001, the unpublished results of which were similar to those reported subsequently by Backman et al.[21]

Bayer's conduct was defended by one of their legal advisers,[25] who pointed out that the FDA had approved the timing of both the change in labelling information proscribing the concomitant use of cerivastatin and gemfibrozil and the subsequent withdrawal of cerivastatin from the market. It is always easy to be wise after the event, but the impression left by these disclosures is that both Bayer and the FDA reacted too slowly to the warning signs of drug toxicity. It was, after all, the FDA that first documented the increased likelihood of rhabdomyolysis from statin–gemfibrozil interaction,[1] eight years before cerivastatin was even launched. For its part, Bayer was at best guilty of adopting an ostrich mentality; at worst of conducting a deliberate cover-up. Either way, cerivastatin was a disastrous and costly failure, in stark contrast to the success enjoyed by other currently marketed statins.

References

1. Thompson GR. Introduction. A symposium: cerivastatin: clinical efficacy and safety in the management of hyperlipidemia. *Am J Cardiol* 1998; **82**(4B): 1J–2J.
2. Pogson GW, Kindred LH, Carper BG. Rhabdomyolysis and renal failure associated with cerivastatin–gemfibrozil combination therapy. *Am J Cardiol* 1999; **83**: 1146.
3. Pierce LR, Wysowski DK, Gross TP. Myopathy and rhabdomyolysis associated with lovastatin–gemfibrozil combination therapy. *JAMA* 1990; **264**: 71–5.
4. Guyton JR, Dujovne CA, Illingworth DR. Dual hepatic metabolism of cerivastatin – clarifications. *Am J Cardiol* 1999; **84**: 497.
5. Ozdemir O, Boran M, Gökçe V, et al. A case with severe rhabdomyolysis and renal failure associated with cerivastatin–gemfibrozil combination therapy – a case report. *Angiology* 2000; **51**: 695–7.
6. Hyman DJ, Henry A, Taylor A. Severe rhabdomyolysis related to cerivastatin without gemfibrozil. *Ann Intern Med* 2002; **137**: 74.
7. Isaacsohn J, Insull W Jr, Stein E, et al. Long-term efficacy and safety of cerivastatin 0.8 mg in patients with primary hypercholesterolemia. *Clin Cardiol* 2001; **24**(9 Suppl): IV1–9.
8. Tuffs A. Bayer faces potential fine over cholesterol lowering drug. *Br Med J* 2001; **323**: 415.
9. Fleck F. Bayer faces Swiss criminal probe over cerivastatin. *Br Med J* 2002; **324**: 130.
10. Marwick C. Bayer is forced to release documents over withdrawal of cerivastatin. *Br Med J* 2003; **326**: 518.
11. Farmer JA. Learning from the cerivastatin experience. *Lancet* 2001; **358**: 1383–4.
12. Staffa JA, Chang J, Green L. Cerivastatin and reports of fatal rhabdomyolysis. *N Engl J Med* 2002; **346**: 539–40.

13. Chang JT, Staffa JA, Parks M, Green L. Rhabdomyolysis with HMG-CoA reductase inhibitors and gemfibrozil combination therapy. *Pharmacoepidemiol Drug Saf* 2004; **13**: 417–26.

14. Graham DJ, Staffa JA, Shatin D, et al. Incidence of hospitalized rhabdomyolysis in patients treated with lipid-lowering drugs. *JAMA* 2004; **292**: 2585–90.

15. Jones PH, Davidson MH. Reporting rate of rhabdomyolysis with fenofibrate + statin versus gemfibrozil + any statin. *Am J Cardiol* 2005; **95**: 120–2.

16. Cholesterol Treatment Trialists' (CTT) Collaborators. Efficacy and safety of cholesterol-lowering treatment: prospective meta-analysis of data from 90,056 participants in 14 randomised trials of statins. *Lancet* 2005; **366**: 1267–78.

17. Thompson PD, Clarkson P, Karas RH. Statin-associated myopathy. *JAMA* 2003; **289**: 1681–90.

18. Nishimoto T, Tozawa R, Amano Y, et al. Comparing myotoxic effects of squalene synthase inhibitor, T-91485, and 3-hydroxy-3-methylglutaryl coenzyme A (HMG-CoA) reductase inhibitors in human myocytes. *Biochem Pharmacol* 2003; **66**: 2133–9.

19. Schaefer WH, Lawrence JW, Loughlin AF, et al. Evaluation of ubiquinone concentration and mitochondrial function relative to cerivastatin-induced skeletal myopathy in rats. *Toxicol Appl Pharmacol* 2004; **194**: 10–23.

20. Johnson TE, Zhang X, Bleicher KB, et al. Statins induce apoptosis in rat and human myotube cultures by inhibiting protein geranylgeranylation but not ubiquinone. *Toxicol Appl Pharmacol* 2004; **200**: 237–50.

21. Backman JT, Kyrklund C, Neuvonen M, Neuvonen PJ. Gemfibrozil greatly increases plasma concentrations of cerivastatin. *Clin Pharmacol Ther* 2002; **72**: 685–91.

22. Prueksaritanont T, Zhao JJ, Ma B, et al. Mechanistic studies on metabolic interactions between gemfibrozil and statins. *J Pharmacol Exp Ther* 2002; **301**: 1042–51.

23. Psaty BM, Furberg CD, Ray WA, Weiss NS. Potential for conflict of interest in the evaluation of suspected adverse drug reactions: use of cerivastatin and risk of rhabdomyolysis. *JAMA* 2004; **292**: 2622–31.

24. Fontanarosa PB, Rennie D, DeAngelis CD. Postmarketing surveillance – lack of vigilance, lack of trust. *JAMA* 2004; **292**: 2647–50.

25. Piorkowski JD Jr. Bayer's response to 'Potential for conflict of interest in the evaluation of suspected adverse drug reactions: use of cerivastatin and risk of rhabdomyolysis'. *JAMA* 2004; **292**: 2655–7.

CHAPTER 11

Phytosterols
Functional or dysfunctional foods?

Chapter summary

- Development of phytosterols as functional foods

- Efficacy and safety of plant sterols and stanols

- Contrasting effects on plasma plant sterols

- Are absorbed plant sterols pro- or anti-atherogenic?

The term 'functional food' entered the vocabulary relatively recently and is defined in the *Concise Oxford Dictionary* as 'a food containing health-giving additives'. By far the best validated of the functional foods claiming to lower cholesterol are those containing plant sterols and stanols, such as the Flora Pro-activ and Benecol products, respectively. Ever since they were introduced, there have been arguments over whether or not these functional foods should be classified as drugs, but European and UK regulatory agencies currently regard them as foods. So, too, does the US Food and Drug Administration (FDA), which accords them GRAS ('generally regarded as safe') status in the USA. Recently, however, concerns have arisen following the publication of research suggesting that plant sterols might have undesirable effects on the cardiovascular system. Other studies have found just the opposite, making this a controversial issue that needs to be resolved.

Plant sterols and stanols, referred to collectively as phytosterols, closely resemble cholesterol structurally; plant sterols, exemplified by sitosterol and campesterol, differ from it only in their side chains, whereas the corresponding plant stanols, sitostanol and campestanol, are saturated sterols and lack a double bond. Phytosterols cannot be synthesized by man, but are present in the diet in cereals, vegetable oils, nuts and seeds, mainly as plant sterol. The dietary intake of the latter is similar to cholesterol, about 300 mg daily, but the concentration of plant sterols in human plasma is <0.5% that of cholesterol, reflecting their poor absorption and lack of endogenous synthesis. The dietary intake of plant stanols is lower, and they are even less well absorbed than plant sterols, with the result that their plasma concentrations are only one-tenth as high – that is, < 0.05% – as that of cholesterol. Fluctuations in very-low-density lipoprotein (VLDL), low-density lipoprotein (LDL) and high-density lipoprotein (HDL), which transport plant sterols and stanols as well as cholesterol, exert an additional influence on plasma levels. To correct for this, the latter are often expressed as ratios to total cholesterol.

Development of phytosterols as functional foods

The cholesterol-lowering properties of plant sterols were first demonstrated in humans over 50 years ago in volunteers given crude sitosterol.[1] Subsequently, it was shown that a commercial preparation of plant sterols derived from soya bean oil lowered patients' cholesterol but markedly increased their plasma level of plant sterols.[2] This raised concerns over safety, inasmuch as the recessively inherited disorder sitosterolaemia, which is characterized by plasma plant sterol concentrations 30 times higher than normal, results in premature atherosclerosis.[3]

The first report of the therapeutic use of plant stanols was in 1986,[4] and it demonstrated that capsules of sitostanol dispersed in sunflower oil lowered LDL cholesterol. However, sitostanol was ineffective in another study, probably because the capsules contained insufficient sunflower oil to solubilize it, and this drew attention to the importance of the physical state of phytosterols as a determinant of efficacy. Application of existing knowledge that the low lipid solubility of sterols may be overcome by esterification led to the development of stanol esters as a means of incorporating plant stanols into food products. This process was patented by the Finnish company Raisio in 1989 and culminated 6 years later in the launch of Benecol margarine. Subsequently, plant sterol esters were incorporated into margarine by Unilever and marketed as Flora Pro-activ.

One of the major sources of the ingredients used in the manufacture of Benecol is tall oil, derived from the pulping of pine wood. Crude tall oil is fractionated into rosin and pitch, the latter containing a mixture of plant stanols and sterols. The plant sterols are catalytically hydrogenated to form stanols and are then esterified with mono- and polyunsaturated fatty acids. Another source of plant sterols is vegetable oil, mainly soya, rapeseed and sunflower. Tall oil pitch is also used in the manufacture of asphalt.

Research into the mechanism of action of plant sterols showed that they lower plasma cholesterol by inhibiting cholesterol absorption, the maximal effect being evident at an intake of 3 g daily. A comparative study revealed that ingestion of plant sterol and stanol esters reduced cholesterol absorption to an equal extent, by about one-third, an effect which is dependent upon hydrolysis of the ester bonds by pancreatic enzymes. The ensuing release of free sterols or stanols displaces cholesterol from mixed micelles within the intestinal lumen, thereby inhibiting the uptake of both dietary and endogenous (mainly biliary) cholesterol.

It is now known that net absorption of cholesterol reflects not just influx from mixed micelles but also its efflux into the intestinal lumen. The latter process is regulated by two ATP-binding cassette (ABC) transporter proteins, ABC G5 and G8, which promote the efflux of roughly half the cholesterol taken up by the intestinal mucosa and nearly all the plant sterol and stanol. Loss-of-function mutations of these transporters results in unregulated absorption of phytosterols and is the cause of sitosterolaemia. Genetic variation at the ABC G5 and G8 loci is responsible also for differences between normal individuals in plasma levels of plant sterols,[5] the latter being regarded as indices of cholesterol absorption.[6] Miettinen et al conducted a subgroup analysis of the Finnish participants of the Scandinavian Simvastatin Survival Study, which showed that subjects with plasma sterol levels indicative of a high rate of cholesterol absorption responded suboptimally to simvastatin, in terms of both LDL-lowering and reduction in coronary events.[7] This may reflect the fact that efficient absorption of cholesterol from the intestine downregulates cholesterol synthesis in the liver, resulting in decreased responsiveness to statins.

Efficacy and safety of plant sterols and stanols

The cholesterol-lowering efficacy and safety of phytosterols have been the subject of a detailed review by Katan et al.[8] This included a meta-analysis of 41 randomized, double-blind trials, of which 20 used plant stanols, 16 used plant sterols, and 5 investigated both. The doses, expressed as free sterol or stanol, ranged from 0.7 to 3.2 g daily and were administered for an average duration of 7 weeks. The mean reduction in LDL cholesterol on plant stanol 2.5 g daily was 10.1%, and it did not differ significantly from that on plant sterol 2.3 g daily, which was 9.7%. However, in two studies, each lasting a year, plant stanol ester in doses of 1.8 and 2.6 g daily reduced LDL cholesterol by 8.5% and by 13%, respectively,[9] whereas plant sterol ester 1.6 g daily lowered it by only 5.9%.[10] The latter result may reflect differences in study design, including the ethnicity of the subjects, background diet, and the fact that the dose of plant sterol used was well below the optimum of 2.5 g daily.[8]

Trials in patients taking statins have shown that consumption of plant sterols or stanols reduce LDL cholesterol by an additional 7–11%, an effect greater than that to be expected from doubling the dose of statin.[11] As regards safety, the only statistically significant change associated with taking phytosterols was a 12% decrease in plasma β-carotene levels, without any decrease in the fat-soluble vitamins A, D or E.[8]

No clinical end-point trials of the use of phytosterols to prevent cardiovascular disease have been undertaken, nor is it likely that they ever will be, in view of the very large number of subjects needed and the huge costs involved. However, by extrapolation from drug trials, a reduction in LDL cholesterol of 10% would be expected to decrease the incidence of cardiovascular disease by 12–20% over the course of 5 years.[8] Based on that premise, the FDA authorized a claim that foods containing either plant sterol or stanol esters may reduce cardiovascular risk. In the UK, the second Joint British Societies' guidelines on the prevention of cardiovascular disease endorsed their use for this purpose in high-risk subjects.

Contrasting effects on plasma plant sterols

As stated previously, the main difference between plant sterols and stanols is their contrasting effect on plasma plant sterols. Consumption of plant sterol esters raises plasma plant sterol levels, especially campesterol,[10] whereas plant stanol esters lower them. These changes are especially marked in patients with familial hypercholesterolaemia taking statins; both the disease itself[11] and these drugs[12] are known to increase plasma plant sterol levels. Evidence of the differential effects of plant sterols and stanols is derived from both population studies[13] and clinical trials. In one such trial, serum sitosterol plus campesterol levels ranged from 0.5 to 2 mg/100 ml at baseline and increased by 35–120% on plant sterol 1.6 g daily,[8] whereas, in another trial, the same amount of plant stanol decreased serum levels of both those plant sterols by 20-40%.[14]

Are absorbed plant sterols pro- or anti-atherogenic?

In view of the atherogenicity of high levels of plant sterols in sitosterolaemia, the question has been raised whether the lesser increases seen in normal subjects taking plant sterols might also be harmful. Specifically, could the potentially cardioprotective, LDL-lowering effect of plant sterols be diminished or counteracted by the accompanying increase in plasma plant sterol levels? If this were to be shown, plant stanols would probably become the preferred adjunct to dietary means of lowering cholesterol. Although consumption of plant stanols increases plasma plant stanol levels,[13] these are normally so low that the likelihood of any toxicity seems minimal.

Epidemiological studies of the association between plasma plant sterols and cardiovascular disease have given ambiguous and confusing results. A nested, case–control analysis of the Prospective Cardiovascular Munster (PROCAM) Study showed that plasma sitosterol concentrations, but not sitosterol:cholesterol ratios, were higher on univariate analysis in cases of coronary heart disease than in controls.[15] The opposite result was seen in the European Prospective Investigation of Cancer (EPIC) Norfolk Population Study, where the plasma sitosterol:cholesterol ratio, but not the sitosterol concentration, was lower in cases of coronary heart disease than in controls.[16] However, the decreased odds ratio for coronary events in those with a sitosterol:cholesterol ratio in the upper tertile was no longer significant after adjustment for traditional risk factors.

The most recent results have come from a nested, case–control study in participants of the Longitudinal Aging Study Amsterdam (LASA), which showed that plant sterol levels and ratios were both significantly lower in subjects who had coronary events than in those who did not.[17] The apparent protection conferred by higher plasma plant sterol levels might perhaps reflect a vegetarian diet and lifestyle, but data on this are lacking. The alternative explanation, that a decreased level of plasma plant sterols predisposes to cardiovascular disease, is hard to envisage in mechanistic terms without invoking hypothetical confounding effects associated with, for example, inheritance of the ABC G8 genotypes that cause low plasma plant sterol levels.[5]

The latest contributions to this controversy have come from groups led by the doyens of research in this field, namely Tatu Miettinen (Figure 11.1) in Helsinki and Klaus von Bergmann in Bonn. The German group measured plant sterols in the plasma and aortic valves of 82 patients having an aortic valve replacement, 10 of whom had been consuming a plant sterol-containing margarine for over 2 years before undergoing surgery.[18] Those who had done so regularly had plasma campesterol levels more than double those of non-users and concentrations of campesterol in the aortic valve cusps fourfold higher. An increase in plasma and aortic valve campesterol was seen also in patients on statins and those with a family history of cardiovascular disease. Overall, there was a strong correlation between plasma and tissue concentrations of plant sterols in this study.

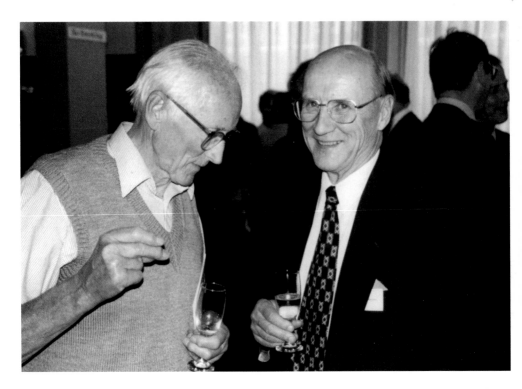

Figure 11.1 *Nick Myant and Tatu Miettinen (right) at the Festschrift meeting for the author held in September 1998 at Hammersmith Hospital (photograph by Frans O'Neill)*

Results from a similar investigation from Finland in which 21 aortic valves were analysed for their plant sterol content were recently published.[19] Two of the patients involved had used a plant sterol-containing margarine, two used a plant stanol-containing margarine, and eight had been on a statin. Once again, there was a strong correlation between campesterol:cholesterol ratios in serum and aortic valves, and serum levels were higher in those on statins, although not in those on phytosterols. The concentrations of cholesterol and campesterol in the valves were strongly correlated, leading the authors to suggest that plant sterols might contribute to aortic stenosis by either promoting inflammation or facilitating the entry of cholesterol.

These findings are of considerable interest but they do not prove that plant sterols are pathogenic per se, or at least not in the concentrations seen in these studies. Although Weingartner et al provided convincing ancillary data obtained in genetically manipulated mice which showed that plant sterols were atherogenic independently of changes in plasma cholesterol,[18] they acknowledged that the amount of plant sterol used in their experiments was 100-fold higher in relative terms than that consumed by humans taking a plant sterol-enriched margarine.

It is intriguing that most of the sterol in the tendon xanthomas and aortas of patients with sitosterolaemia is cholesterol, not plant sterol,[20] despite their relatively normal levels of serum cholesterol. This supports the suggestion that plant sterols somehow promote cholesterol deposition.[19] Analysis of carotid plaques in normal subjects has shown that the percentage of free campesterol is higher than that of free cholesterol,[21] supporting observations that its esterification and clearance by macrophages is slower.[22] This, together with the finding in sitosterolaemia that the tissue-to-plasma ratio of plant sterols is higher than that of cholesterol, suggests that they accumulate more readily in the arterial wall. Nevertheless, it must be stressed that the concentration of plant sterols in the aortic plaques of normal individuals is still 100-fold less than that of cholesterol.[23]

This leaves a number of questions still to be answered. Does a doubling of the plasma plant sterol level either predispose to or protect against coronary heart disease? Is the presence of plant sterols in aortic valves and atheromatous plaques[21] simply a marker of LDL deposition or is it evidence of atherogenicity? If the latter applies, to what extent might this offset the LDL-lowering benefits of plant sterols? More research is needed before these issues can be resolved, but it is important that they should be, not least for the future well-being of those consuming plant sterol-enriched foods.

References

1. Pollak OJ. Reduction of blood cholesterol in man. *Circulation* 1953; **7**: 702–6.
2. Lees RS, Lees AM. Effects of sitosterol therapy on plasma lipid and lipoprotein concentrations. In Greten H, ed. *Lipoprotein Metabolism.* Berlin: Springer-Verlag, 1976: 119–24.
3. Bhattacharyya AK, Connor WE. β-Sitosterolemia and xanthomatosis. A newly described lipid storage disease in two sisters. *J Clin Invest* 1974; **53**: 1033–43.
4. Heinemann T, Leiss O, von Bergmann K. Effect of low-dose sitostanol on serum cholesterol in patients with hypercholesterolemia. *Atherosclerosis* 1986; **61**: 219–23.
5. Berg KE, von Bergmann K, Lutjohann D, et al. Heritability of plasma noncholesterol sterols and relationship to DNA sequence polymorphism in ABCG5 and ABCG8. *J Lipid Res* 2002; **43**: 486–94.
6. Miettinen TA, Tilvis RS, Kesaniemi YA. Serum plant sterols and cholesterol precursors reflect cholesterol absorption and synthesis in volunteers of a randomly selected male population. *Am J Epidemiol* 1990; **131**: 20–31.
7. Miettinen TA, Strandberg TE, Gylling H, for the Finnish Investigators of the Scandinavian Simvastatin Survival Study Group. Non-cholesterol sterols and cholesterol lowering by long-term simvastatin treatment in coronary patients. *Arterioscler Thromb Vasc Biol* 2000; **20**: 1340–6.

8. Katan MB, Grundy SM, Jones P, et al. Efficacy and safety of plant stanols and sterols in the management of blood cholesterol levels. *Mayo Clin Proc* 2003; **78**: 965–78.

9. Miettinen TA, Puska P, Gylling H, et al. Reduction of serum cholesterol with sitostanol-ester margarine in a mildly hyper-cholesterolemic population. *N Engl J Med* 1995; **333**: 1308–12.

10. Hendriks HF, Brink EJ, Meijer GW, et al. Safety of long-term consumption of plant sterol esters-enriched spread. *Eur J Clin Nutr* 2003; **57**: 681–92.

11. Thompson GR. Additive effects of plant sterol and stanol esters to statin therapy. *Am J Cardiol* 2005; **96**(Suppl): 37D–39D.

12. Miettinen TA, Gylling H, Lindbohm N, et al. Serum noncholesterol sterols during inhibition of cholesterol synthesis by statins. *J Lab Clin Med* 2003; **141**: 131–7.

13. Fransen HP, de Jong N, Wolfs M, et al. Customary use of plant sterol and stanol enriched margarine is associated with changes in serum plant sterol and stanol concentrations in humans. *J Nutr* 2007; **137**: 1301–6.

14. O'Neill FH, Sanders TA, Thompson GR. Comparison of efficacy of plant stanol ester and sterol ester: short-term and longer-term studies. *Am J Cardiol* 2005; **96**(Suppl): 29D–36D.

15. Assmann G, Cullen P, Erbey J, et al. Plasma sitosterol elevations are associated with an increased incidence of coronary events in men: results of a nested case–control analysis of the Prospective Cardiovascular Munster (PROCAM) Study. *Nutr Metab Cardiovasc Dis* 2006; **16**: 13–21.

16. Pinedo S, Vissers MN, von Bergmann K, et al. Plasma levels of plant sterols and the risk of coronary artery disease: the prospective EPIC-Norfolk Population Study. *J Lipid Res* 2007; **48**: 139–44.

17. Fassbender K, Lutjohann D, Dik MG, et al. Moderately elevated plant sterol levels are associated with reduced cardiovascular risk – the LASA study. *Atherosclerosis* 2008; **196**: 283–8.

18. Weingartner O, Lutjohann D, Ji S, et al. Vascular effects of diet supplementation with plant sterols. *J Am Coll Cardiol* 2008; **51**: 1553–61.

19. Helske S, Miettinen T, Gylling H, et al. Accumulation of cholesterol precursors and plant sterols in human aortic valves. *J Lipid Res* 2008; 8 April 2008 (Epub ahead of print).

20. Salen G, Horak I, Rothkopf M, et al. Lethal atherosclerosis associated with abnormal plasma and tissue sterol composition in sitosterolemia with xanthomatosis. *J Lipid Res* 1985; **26**: 1126–33.

21. Miettinen TA, Railo M, Lepantalo M, Gylling H. Plant sterols in serum and in atherosclerotic plaques of patients undergoing carotid endarterectomy. *J Am Coll Cardiol* 2005; **45**: 1794–801.

22. Sato Y, Nishikawa K, Aikawa K, et al. Side-chain structure is critical for the transport of sterols from lysosomes to cytoplasm. *Biochim Biophys Acta* 1995; **1257**: 38–46.

23. Mellies MJ, Ishikawa TT, Glueck CK, et al. Phytosterols in aortic tissue in adults and infants. *J Lab Clin Med* 1976; **88**: 914–21.

CHAPTER 12

The continuing controversy over cholesterol-regulating drugs

Unexpected outcome of trials of ezetimibe and torcetrapib

The lipid hypothesis may have been laid to rest by the statin trials, but cholesterol remains a controversial topic, especially when the pharmaceutical industry is involved. This was exemplified by the publicity generated recently by the negative outcome of clinical trials of two novel cholesterol-regulating drugs, torcetrapib and ezetimibe. Before discussing the issues involved, the mechanism of action of these drugs must first be considered, and that, in turn, requires a rudimentary knowledge of cholesterol metabolism. Lipidologists will probably regard the following description as simplistic, but others might find it helpful.

Cholesterol metabolism

Cholesterol plays an essential physiological role, and its metabolism is closely regulated by enzymes, receptors and transfer proteins located in the small intestine, liver, peripheral cells (including those lining the arterial wall) and plasma (Figure 12.1). After hepatic synthesis or intestinal absorption, cholesterol is esterified with fatty acids in the liver and then secreted, together with triglyceride, into plasma in the form of very-low-density lipoprotein (VLDL) particles. The latter are rapidly converted into low-density lipoprotein (LDL) particles, which circulate in the blood for several days before binding to LDL receptors on liver cells. Some of the cholesterol returning to the liver in this manner is then excreted in the bile, either unchanged

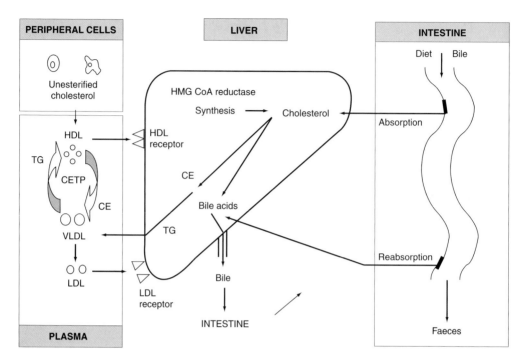

Figure 12.1 *Schematic diagram of cholesterol metabolism (CE: cholesterol ester; CETP: cholesterol ester transfer protein; TG: triglyceride) (reproduced with permission from Thompson G, Morrell J, Wilson P. Dyslipidaemia in Clinical Practice (2nd edn). London: Informa Healthcare, 2006)*

or after conversion into bile acids, and the remainder is resecreted as VLDL. Factors which enhance production or diminish excretion increase the amount of LDL cholesterol in plasma. This can then accumulate in the arterial wall and promote atherosclerosis – hence its synonym, 'bad cholesterol'.

The function of high-density lipoprotein (HDL) particles is to promote the efflux of unesterified cholesterol from peripheral cells and transport it back into plasma for eventual disposal in the liver, a process termed 'reverse cholesterol transport'. This recycling role, together with epidemiological evidence that the concentration of HDL cholesterol in plasma is inversely correlated with the risk of coronary heart disease, has given rise to the synonym 'good cholesterol'. Reverse cholesterol transport involves the esterification and subsequent exchange of cholesterol in HDL for triglyceride in VLDL, a process mediated in plasma by cholesterol ester transfer protein (CETP) (Figure 12.1). Genetic lack or pharmacological inhibition of CETP interrupts the exchange process, causing cholesterol to accumulate in HDL and increasing its concentration in plasma.

Evidence for the atherogenic effect of LDL is much stronger than that for the protective properties of HDL. Hence, most forms of therapy aimed at preventing atherosclerosis have focused on lowering LDL, the most successful being the statin class of drugs. By inhibiting the enzyme hydroxymethylglutaryl co-enzyme A (HMG CoA) reductase, these drugs reduce cholesterol synthesis; this decreases VLDL secretion and increases the expression of LDL receptors in the liver, thereby enhancing the rate of removal of LDL from plasma. In the Cholesterol Treatment Trialists' Collaborators' meta-analysis, the mean reduction in LDL cholesterol in subjects on statins was 29%, which was associated with a 21% decrease in coronary mortality.[1] It was suggested that decreasing LDL cholesterol by 50%, achievable with high doses of atorvastatin and rosuvastatin, could reduce the risk of coronary disease by 40%. However, this would still leave at risk the majority of those on treatment – and this brings us back to ezetimibe and torcetrapib and the rationale behind their development.

Ezetimibe

Ezetimibe acts like phytosterols by inhibiting the intestinal absorption of cholesterol derived from biliary and dietary sources. Unlike phytosterols, it does not affect micellar solubilization but binds to and inhibits the Niemann-Pick C1-like 1 protein that mediates intestinal uptake of cholesterol from mixed micelles. The ensuing reduction in LDL cholesterol is additive to the effect of statins; combining ezetimibe with a statin augments the latter's LDL-lowering efficacy by a further 15–20% and would be expected to achieve a correspondingly greater reduction in risk of coronary heart disease than the statin alone. For example, the combination of rosuvastatin and ezetimibe has been shown to reduce LDL cholesterol by almost 70%,[2] and this, in theory, could halve the risk of coronary heart disease. Clinical outcome trials of ezetimibe to test this premise are currently in progress, but in the meantime controversy has arisen over the results of the ENHANCE study, which compared the effects of simvastatin with those of simvastatin plus ezetimibe on a surrogate marker of atherosclerosis.

The ENHANCE trial was a double-blind, multicentre study which compared the anti-atherosclerotic effects of simvastatin 80 mg and simvastatin 80 mg plus ezetimibe 10 mg daily in over 600 patients with heterozygous familial hypercholesterolaemia (FH).[3] The primary end point was change in carotid intima-medial thickness (IMT) after 2 years, as measured by ultrasound. The results reveal that LDL cholesterol values were reduced by 41% by simvastatin versus 58% by simvastatin and ezetimibe combined. Baseline values of carotid IMT were surprisingly normal for patients with FH and presumably reflect the fact that 80% had been on lipid-lowering therapy prior to the study, which would tend to reverse any previous accumulation of cholesterol in the vessel wall.[4]

During the study, IMT increased by 0.0058 mm on simvastatin and by 0.0111 mm on combination therapy, but the difference between the treatment groups was not significant. This raises the question of whether the apparent lack of benefit from ezetimibe in ENHANCE was due to the fact that, despite the greater reduction in LDL cholesterol in those on simvastatin plus ezetimibe, it lowers LDL by a different mechanism from statins and therefore lacks their pleiotropic effects. The latter include improved endothelial function and anti-inflammatory properties. However, it is debatable whether these actions are genuinely independent of the LDL-lowering effect of statins and, if so, whether they make any additional contribution to the reduction in clinical events.[5] A meta-analysis that compared trials conducted in the pre-statin era, using diet, bile acid sequestrants and partial ileal bypass, with trials using statins showed that in both instances the reduction in cardiovascular risk was directly proportional to the extent of reduction of LDL cholesterol.[6] In other words, the pleiotropic effects of statins did not appear to contribute any additional benefit.

Bile acid sequestrants and ezetimibe both upregulate HMG CoA reductase, so neither can exert the LDL-independent, pleiotropic effects attributed to statins, which reflect inhibition of HMG CoA reductase. Hence, the argument that the negative outcome of ENHANCE was due to the lack of these pleiotropic effects lacks credibility. So, too, do calls to withdraw or withhold ezetimibe from patients, especially since there was no increase in adverse events when it was combined with simvastatin. Clearly, the results of a large clinical outcome trial now under way (IMPROVE-IT) are needed before this controversial issue can be resolved, but that will not be until 2011.[7] Until then, achieving LDL cholesterol targets remains a valid strategy in which ezetimibe can play an important role when other approaches have failed.

Torcetrapib

To turn now to consider torcetrapib; the short history of this ill-fated compound epitomizes TH Huxley's epigram 'the great tragedy of science – the staying of a beautiful hypothesis by an ugly fact'. The beautiful hypothesis was that increasing HDL cholesterol by means of a CETP inhibitor would reduce the risk of coronary heart disease; the ugly fact was that the CETP inhibitor used for this purpose, torcetrapib increased overall mortality from cardiovascular and other causes by almost 60% within the course of 1 year.

Evidence that raised levels of HDL cholesterol are inversely correlated with the incidence of coronary heart disease and associated with longevity implies that inherited or acquired increases in HDL would be protective. A recent study showed that almost 40% of the variation in HDL cholesterol between individuals is genetically determined, a quarter of which is attributable to polymorphisms of the CETP gene.[8] Lifestyle factors which decrease CETP activity and thereby raise HDL cholesterol include alcohol consumption, which accounts for half of the environmental variation in HDL seen in men.[9,10] Since moderate consumption of alcohol is known to be associated with some degree of protection against coronary heart disease, this suggests that reduction of CETP activity would be a valid therapeutic objective.

Several CETP gene mutations decrease CETP activity and raise HDL, but the evidence that they are indeed beneficial is conflicting. On the positive side, a highly significant increase in the frequency of a mutation associated with reduced CETP activity has been found in Ashkenazi Jews with exceptional longevity.[11] The Framingham Offspring Study found that another common CETP polymorphism conferred a reduced risk of coronary heart disease in men (but not women) and the same also applied in the Veterans Affairs HDL Cholesterol Intervention Trial (VA-HIT).[12] In contrast, a CETP mutation associated with markedly raised levels of HDL cholesterol in northern Japan was found to be less frequent after the age of 80,[13] and an increased prevalence of coronary heart disease was seen in men of Japanese ancestry[14] and Danish women (but not men) with other CETP mutations.[15]

The conflicting evidence makes it hard to decide whether genetically determined decreases in CETP are protective or hazardous to health. The beneficial effects of CETP deficiency have been attributed to the accompanying elevation of HDL cholesterol, and the adverse effects to impaired reverse cholesterol transport resulting in a loss of the anti-atherogenic properties of HDL particles consequent on their increased cholesterol content and size. The recent development of CETP inhibitors seems to offer an ideal means of settling this issue.

The clinical potential of torcetrapib was first reported in 2004, based on a small study of patients with low HDL cholesterol levels, half of whom were taking atorvastatin.[16] Torcetrapib 120 mg daily increased HDL cholesterol by 61% in patients on atorvastatin and by 46% in those on torcetrapib alone, these changes being due to 30–40% decreases in plasma CETP activity. Similar results were observed in two larger trials in subjects with below-average values of HDL cholesterol given torcetrapib 10–90 mg daily. Increases in blood pressure were noted in 2 of 140 subjects given torcetrapib alone[17] and in 4 of 137 subjects on torcetrapib plus atorvastatin,[18] but otherwise the drug was well tolerated.

Against this background, three larger trials of torcetrapib were conducted in 2005/06. RADIANCE 1 investigated the effect of atorvastatin with and without torcetrapib 60 mg daily in 850 patients with FH, using ultrasound to measure changes in carotid IMT.[19] ILLUSTRATE investigated the effects of atorvastatin with and without torcetrapib 60 mg daily in almost 1200 patients with coronary disease, using intravascular ultrasound to assess progression of coronary atherosclerosis.[20] ILLUMINATE, the largest of the three trials, compared the effects of atorvastatin with those of atorvastatin plus torcetrapib 60 mg/day on the frequency of cardiovascular events in over 15 000 high-risk subjects.[21]

The results of RADIANCE 1 showed the expected increase in HDL cholesterol in FH subjects on atorvastatin plus torcetrapib and an additional decrease in LDL cholesterol compared with those on atorvastatin alone. The primary end point, increase in maximum carotid IMT, did not differ between the treatment groups after 2 years, but the increase in mean carotid IMT/year, a secondary end point, was significantly greater in those on atorvastatin plus torcetrapib. Subjects in this group also showed a 3-mm increase in systolic blood pressure and sustained twice as many cardiovascular events as did those on atorvastatin alone.

Similar changes in serum lipids were seen in ILLUSTRATE, with a 60% increase in HDL cholesterol and a 20% decrease in LDL cholesterol in patients on atorvastatin plus torcetrapib compared with those on atorvastatin alone. There was no difference in the extent to which coronary atherosclerosis progressed in the two treatment groups over the course of 2 years, but systolic blood pressure increased by 4.6 mm in patients on combination therapy.

The ILLUMINATE trial began randomizing patients in mid-2004 and was due to last for 4.5 years. However, the trial was stopped abruptly in December 2006 by the manufacturers of torcetrapib, Pfizer, on account of a 58% increase in total mortality after 1 year in patients taking atorvastatin plus torcetrapib compared with those on atorvastatin alone. This reflected increases in both cardiovascular and non-cardiovascular causes of death. Patients on combination therapy had a 4.5-mm greater rise in systolic blood pressure than those on atorvastatin monotherapy, together with accompanying changes in serum electrolytes suggestive of increased aldosterone activity.

The future of CETP inhibitors

The disastrous outcome of ILLUMINATE inevitably led to much heart searching concerning the factors responsible. One possible explanation for the increase in cardiovascular deaths was the increase in blood pressure associated with torcetrapib, which arguably could be a specific side-effect of this compound rather than of CETP inhibitors in general. Alternatively, it might be that inhibition of CETP is intrinsically atherogenic, presumably because it impairs reverse cholesterol transport in plasma.

Whatever the explanation, the results of RADIANCE 1, ILLUS-TRATE and ILLUMINATE sounded the death knell for torce-trapib, although not necessarily for all CETP inhibitors. Another of these compounds, anacetrapib, has been shown recently to induce even greater increases in HDL cholesterol and decreases in LDL cholesterol than torcetrapib but without increasing blood pressure.[22] Further data are urgently needed, including the effects of anacetrapib on surrogate markers of atherosclerosis and on clinical outcome, in order to determine whether there is any future for CETP inhibitors in the prevention of cardiovascular disease.

References

1. Cholesterol Treatment Trialists' (CTT) Collaborators. Efficacy and safety of cholesterol-lowering treatment: prospective meta-analysis of data from 90,056 participants in 14 randomised trials of statins. *Lancet* 2005; **366**; 1267–78.
2. Ballantyne CM, Weiss R, Moccetti T, et al. Efficacy and safety of rosuvastatin 40 mg alone or in combination with ezetimibe in patients at high risk of cardiovascular disease (results from the EXPLORER study). *Am J Cardiol* 2007; **99**: 673–80.
3. Kastelein JJP, Akdim F, Stroes ESG, et al. Simvastatin with or without ezetimibe in familial hypercholesterolemia. *N Engl J Med* 2008; **358**: 1431–43.
4. Brown BG, Taylor AJ. Does ENHANCE diminish confidence in lowering LDL or ezetimibe? *N Engl J Med* 2008; **358**: 1504–7.
5. Futterman LG, Lemberg L. Statin pleiotropy: fact or fiction? *Am J Crit Care* 2004; **13**: 244–9.
6. Robinson JG, Smith B, Maheshwari N, Schrott H. Pleiotropic effects of statins: benefit beyond cholesterol reduction? A meta-regression analysis. *J Am Coll Cardiol* 2005; **46**: 1855–62.
7. Drazen JM, Jarcho JA, Morrissey S, Curfman GD. Cholesterol lowering and ezetimibe. *N Engl J Med* 2008; **358**: 1507–8.
8. Knoblauch H, Bauerfeind A, Toliat MR, et al. Haplotypes and SNPs in 13 lipid-relevant genes explain most of the genetic variance in high-density lipoprotein and low-density lipoprotein cholesterol. *Hum Mol Genet* 2004; **13**: 993–1004.

9. Hannuksela M, Marcel YL, Kesaniemi YA, Savolainen MJ. Reduction in the concentration and activity of plasma cholesterol ester transfer protein by alcohol. *J Lipid Res* 1992; **33**: 737–44.
10. Ellison RC, Zhang Y, Qureshi MM, et al. Investigators of the NHLBI Family Heart Study. Lifestyle determinants of high-density lipoprotein cholesterol: the National Heart, Lung, and Blood Institute Family Heart Study. *Am Heart J* 2004; **147**: 529–35.
11. Barzilai N, Atzmon G, Schechter C, et al. Unique lipoprotein phenotype and genotype associated with exceptional longevity. *JAMA* 2003; **290**: 2030–40.
12. Brousseau ME, O'Connor JJ Jr, Ordovas JM, et al. Cholesteryl ester transfer protein TaqI B2B2 genotype is associated with higher HDL cholesterol levels and lower risk of coronary heart disease end points in men with HDL deficiency. Veterans Affairs HDL Cholesterol Intervention Trial. *Arterioscler Thromb Vasc Biol* 2002; **22**: 1148–54.
13. Hirano K, Yamashita S, Nakajima N, et al. Genetic cholesteryl ester transfer protein deficiency is extremely frequent in the Omagari area of Japan. Marked hyperalphalipoproteinemia caused by CETP gene mutation is not associated with longevity. *Arterioscler Thromb Vasc Biol* 1997; **17**: 1053–9.
14. Zhong S, Sharp DS, Grove JS, et al. Increased coronary heart disease in Japanese-American men with mutation in the cholesteryl ester transfer protein gene despite increased HDL levels. *J Clin Invest* 1996; **97**: 2917–23.
15. Agerholm-Larsen B, Nordestgaard BG, Steffensen R, et al. Elevated HDL cholesterol is a risk factor for ischemic heart disease in white women when caused by a common mutation in the cholesteryl ester transfer protein gene. *Circulation* 2000; **101**: 1907–12.
16. Brousseau ME, Schaefer EJ, Wolfe ML, et al. Effects of an inhibitor of cholesteryl ester transfer protein on HDL cholesterol. *N Engl J Med* 2004; **350**: 1505–15.
17. Davidson MH, McKenney JM, Shear CL, Revkin JH. Efficacy and safety of torcetrapib, a novel cholesteryl ester transfer protein inhibitor, in individuals with below-average high-density lipoprotein cholesterol levels. *J Am Coll Cardiol* 2006; **48**: 1774–81.
18. McKenney JM, Davidson MH, Shear CL, Revkin JH. Efficacy and safety of torcetrapib, a novel cholesteryl ester transfer protein inhibitor, in individuals with below-average high-density lipoprotein cholesterol levels on a background of atorvastatin. *J Am Coll Cardiol* 2006; **48**: 1782–90.
19. Kastelein JJ, van Leuven SI, Burgess L, et al. Effect of torcetrapib on carotid atherosclerosis in familial hypercholesterolemia. *N Engl J Med* 2007; **56**: 1620–30.
20. Nissen SE, Tardif JC, Nicholls SJ, et al. Effect of torcetrapib on the progression of coronary atherosclerosis. *N Engl J Med* 2007; **356**: 1304–16.
21. Barter PJ, Caulfield M, Eriksson M, et al. Effects of torcetrapib in patients at high risk for coronary events. *N Engl J Med* 2007; **357**: 2109–22.

22. Krishna R, Anderson MS, Bergman AJ, et al. Effect of the cholesteryl ester transfer protein inhibitor, anacetrapib, on lipoproteins in patients with dyslipidemia and on 24-h ambulatory blood pressure in healthy individuals: two double-blind, randomised placebo-controlled phase 1 studies. *Lancet* 2007; **370**: 1882–3.

CHAPTER 13

Current trends in cardiovascular disease

Falling mortality rates in Britain reflect changes in treatment and risk factors

Approximately 50 million people are estimated to die in the world each year. In 1990, 28 million of those deaths were due to non-communicable diseases, more than 10 million of which were caused by coronary heart disease and stroke.[1] The expectation is that by 2020 worldwide mortality from non-communicable diseases will have increased by 80%, with cardiovascular disease remaining as the leading cause of death.[2] Hence, it appears that the reduction in cardiovascular mortality now evident in developed countries will be offset by an increase in developing countries, resulting from their adopting the atherogenic Western lifestyle that seemingly is an inevitable accompaniment of economic improvement.

UK statistics

Comparative statistics in Britain[3] are on a smaller scale but similar in relative terms. Total mortality in the UK is approximately 600 000 annually, 36% of which is due to cardiovascular disease. Half of the latter is from coronary heart disease and a quarter from stroke, and cardiovascular disease is the main cause of premature mortality (under 75 years) in both men and women. Coronary mortality peaked in 1970 and has fallen gradually since, decreasing in England and Wales between 1981 and 2000 in men and women by 62% and 45%, respectively. Figure 13.1 shows the decline in England. There has also been a 23% reduction in deaths from stroke before the age of 65 over the past 10 years.

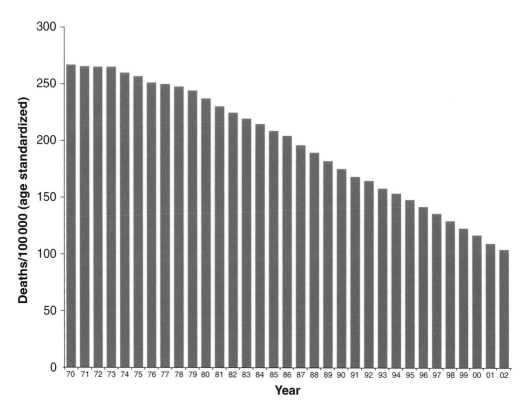

Figure 13.1 *Fall in death rate from coronary heart disease, stroke and other diseases of the circulatory system in people below the age of 75 in England between 1970 and 2002 (reproduced from British Heart Foundation (BHF) coronary heart disease statistics at www.heartstats.org)*

In contrast with mortality, morbidity from coronary heart disease and stroke rose in Britain between 1994 and 2003, prevalence rates increasing by 28% in men and 21% in women. The incidence of myocardial infarction and new cases of angina is currently 227 000 and 95 000, respectively, with corresponding prevalence rates of approximately 1 million each. Overall, it is estimated that coronary heart disease affects more than 2.5 million people in the UK, the highest prevalence being in Scotland, where it affects 8% of men and 6% of women.

The increase in morbidity from cardiovascular disease in Britain partly reflects the decrease in mortality, in that substitution of non-fatal for fatal events contributes to the prevalence of coronary disease. Another factor is the increased life expectancy of the population, inasmuch as the frequency of cardiovascular disease is greatest after the age of 75. In contrast, data from the World Health Organization's MONICA project show that coronary event rates are falling in men and women below the age of 65.[4]

Changes in risk factors and treatment

It has been estimated that the major modifiable risk factors, namely raised serum cholesterol, smoking and high blood pressure, account for 45%, 29% and 22%, respectively, of all myocardial infarcts in Western Europe.[5] Hence, it is important to examine temporal changes in these risk factors when trying to explain shifts in cardiovascular morbidity and mortality. In England in 2003, mean levels of serum total and HDL cholesterol were 5.5 and 1.4 mmol/l in men, and 5.6 and 1.6 mmol/l in women. The percentage of men and women respectively with a total cholesterol >5 mmol/l was lower in 2003 (70.1% and 70.8%) than in 1994 (74.5 and 76.5%). During the same period, the percentages of dietary energy derived from total and saturated fat both decreased (from 37.4% to 36.7% and from 14.9% to 14.5%, respectively). Although these intakes are above those recommended by the Department of Health[6] (total fat under 35%; saturated fat under 10%), they are a considerable improvement on the corresponding values in 1975 (40.4% and 19.3%).

Just under a quarter of British adults smoked in 2005, compared with 42% in 1976 and 28% in 1996. Hence, the rapid rate of decline in smoking during the 1980s slowed considerably after 1990. Mean systolic blood pressure fell by 5 mm in men and 8 mm in women between 1993 and 2005, but roughly one-third of adults in England remain hypertensive.

Thus, changes in the three major risk factors during the past decade have been relatively modest, the prevalence of hyper-cholesterolaemia in men and women decreasing by 6% and 7.5%, smoking by 14% and 18%, and hypertension by 5% and 12%, respectively.

Changes in the treatment of cardiovascular disease over the same period have been far more marked than changes in risk factors. Although coronary artery bypass graft procedures increased by only 15%, the number of percutaneous coronary interventions more than tripled. Prescriptions for anti-hypertensive and anti-platelet drugs increased from four- to fivefold between 1994 and 2005, while prescriptions for lipid-regulating drugs, mainly statins, increased by a staggering 2000%.

In an attempt to explain the 50% decrease in coronary mortality in England and Wales between 1981 and 2000, the number of deaths prevented or postponed by specific cardiac interventions and by risk factor changes has been calculated for each of those years.[7] The results suggest that approximately 42% of the decrease was due to cardiological procedures, both medical and surgical, and the remainder to reductions in cardiovascular risk factors. Of the latter, 48% was due to decreased smoking and 10% each to decreases in cholesterol and blood pressure. The large effect of decreased smoking reflects the fact that its prevalence in Britain fell by almost 40% during the period under analysis.

Subsequently, a similar study was performed to explain the decrease in coronary mortality in the USA over the same period.[8] As in Britain, just under 50% of the reduction in mortality was attributable to medical or surgical interventions, and the remainder reflected risk factor changes. In contrast with Britain, decreased smoking accounted for only 12% of the reduction in coronary mortality, whereas reductions in serum cholesterol and blood pressure contributed to 24% and 20%, respectively. The finding that statins made a much larger contribution to the impact of treatment on coronary heart disease mortality in the USA than in Britain (8.5% vs 0.9%) presumably reflects their greater usage there. However, the prescription rate for these drugs tripled in England in the 5 years following the period surveyed, a fact that should narrow the gap between the UK and US results if the analyses were to be repeated now. Interestingly, a survey of more than 1000 patients with familial hypercholesterolaemia in the UK showed that their mortality from coronary heart disease had halved since 1992, arguably reflecting the universal use of statins to treat such patients after 1989, when simvastatin was first licensed in Britain.[9]

Costs of cardiovascular disease and treatment

Cardiovascular disease and its treatment have an enormous impact on the economy. It is estimated that cardiovascular disease costs the UK £26 billion a year. Of this, 57% is direct health-care costs, 19% is the cost of informal care of those affected, and 24% results from lost productivity.[3] Direct health-care costs mainly reflect inpatient costs (76%) and medications (18%). Lipid-regulating drugs cost the National Health Service (NHS) £625 million in 2005, of which around £600 million was spent on statins. Currently, about 2 million people take statins in England and Wales, but this is projected to rise to over 3 million when recent guidance from the National Institute for Health and Clinical Excellence (NICE)[10] is adopted by general practitioners.

The cost-effectiveness of statins has recently been reviewed by NICE,[11] which deems interventions with a cost of up to £20 000 per quality-adjusted life year (QALY) as cost-effective while those costing £20000–£30000 per QALY are regarded as borderline. Secondary prevention of coronary heart disease with statins carries an incremental cost per QALY of £10000–£16000 and is therefore considered cost-effective. The cost of primary prevention is £10000–£111000 and is heavily influenced by the degree of risk and the age at which treatment is started, being lower at high levels of risk and in younger subjects (those under 45 years of age). In its recent guidance, NICE recommended that the cardiovascular disease risk level for primary prevention with statins should be 20% per 10 years, equivalent to a coronary heart disease risk of 15% per 10 years.

The potential economic benefits of statins in secondary prevention are illustrated by an analysis based on the results of the Scandinavian Simvastatin Survival Study.[12] This showed that the number of days spent in hospital by subjects taking simvastatin was one-third less than by those on placebo, which offset almost 90% of the cost of the drug. As noted earlier, the costs of inpatient treatment far exceed those of medications in the NHS; a similar but more recent analysis of the Heart Protection Study showed that simvastatin reduced the hospitalization costs of vascular events by 22%.[13] The fact that simvastatin is now a generic drug means that it is cheaper and therefore even more cost-effective.

The place of cholesterol-lowering interventions

There is now general acceptance that lipid hypothesis-based preventive strategies for cardiovascular disease are scientifically valid and have proved to be effective in young and middle-aged subjects at high risk. Whether statins should be used across a much wider spectrum of ages and risk categories is more contentious. Not only does their cost-efficacy diminish with increasing age, but doubts have been cast on the ethics of treating the elderly with these drugs. There is a paucity of evidence that statins reduce total mortality after the age of 70, as was illustrated by the PROSPER study,[14] and it has been suggested that their use after this age risks substituting a 'less desirable' death from cancer for a 'more desirable' death from coronary heart disease, albeit at an earlier age. However, no increase in cancer deaths in subjects treated with simvastatin was found by the Heart Protection Study, although just as many participants in that trial were over the age of 70 as in the PROSPER study.[15]

Myant has observed that it is difficult not to feel strongly about the link thought to exist between cholesterol and a disorder as serious and widespread as coronary heart disease, and that it arouses emotions which tend to cloud judgement.[16] This is particularly so when the proposed remedies include the need for large sections of the population to change the habits of a lifetime. An analogous reaction is commonly provoked by the perception that large profits are made by the pharmaceutical industry. For example, the two best-selling drugs in 2004 in the USA were statins, and sales of the latter exceeded $15 billion.[17] In an effort to reduce the huge costs involved, government and consumer organizations in the US and UK are putting pressure on healthcare providers to prescribe generic statins whenever possible. For their part, drug companies fight to preserve their patent rights and point out the high cost of drug development, which has been estimated at $800 million for each new compound which reaches the market.[18]

Despite the caveats about lipid-regulating drugs, as discussed in previous chapters, most people now accept the premise that lowering cholesterol is essential if atherosclerosis and cardiovascular disease are to be prevented. The downward trend in cardiovascular mortality in Britain and other Western countries suggests that this process is now well under way, providing strong support for the lipid hypothesis.

Epilogue

Although the controversy over cholesterol may have died down, it is clearly not yet over. As Francis Bacon pointed out over 400 years ago, 'If a man will begin with certainties, he shall end in doubts; but if he will be content to begin with doubts, he shall end in certainties.'[19] However, there will always be some who begin with doubts and never relinquish them, as epitomized by the International Network of Cholesterol Skeptics. Their motto, 'The growth of knowledge depends entirely on disagreement', recalls the atmosphere of the post-war Hammersmith, where the cholesterol controversy first started in Britain. Sixty years on, it is still flourishing.

References

1. Murray CJ, Lopez AD. Mortality by cause for eight regions of the world: Global Burden of Disease Study. *Lancet* 1997; **349**: 1269–76.
2. Murray CJ, Lopez AD. Alternative projections of mortality and disability by cause 1990–2020: Global Burden of Disease Study. *Lancet* 1997; **349**: 1498–504.
3. Coronary heart disease statistics, 2007 edition. British Heart Foundation Statistics Database. Available at: www.heartstats.org.

4. Tunstall-Pedoe H, Kuulasmaa K, Mahonen M, et al. Contribution of trends in survival and coronary-event rates to changes in coronary heart disease mortality: 10-year results from 37 WHO MONICA Project populations. *Lancet* 1999; **353**: 1547–57.

5. Yusuf S, Hawken S, Ounpuu S, et al. Effect of potentially modifiable risk factors associated with myocardial infarction in 52 countries (the INTERHEART study): case–control study. *Lancet* 2004; **364**: 937–52.

6. Department of Health and Social Security. *Diet and Cardiovascular Disease: Report of the Panel on Diet in Relation to Cardiovascular Disease, Committee on Medical Aspects of Food Policy.* London: HMSO, 1984 (Report on Health and Social Subjects, no. 28).

7. Unal B, Critchley JA, Capewell S. Explaining the decline in coronary heart disease mortality in England and Wales between 1981 and 2000. *Circulation* 2004; **109**: 1101–7.

8. Ford ES, Ajani UA, Croft JB, et al. Explaining the decline in U.S. deaths from coronary disease, 1980–2000. *N Engl J Med* 2007; **356**: 2388–98.

9. Scientific Steering Committee on behalf of the Simon Broome Register Group. Mortality in treated heterozygous familial hypercholesterolaemia: implications for clinical management. *Atherosclerosis* 1999; **142**: 105–12.

10. National Institute for Health and Clinical Excellence. *Lipid modification: cardiovascular risk assessment and the modification of blood lipids for the primary and secondary prevention of cardiovascular disease. NICE clinical guideline 67.* London: NICE, 2008.

11. National Institute for Health and Clinical Excellence. Technology appraisal 94, 2006. Available at: http://guidance.nice.org.uk/TA94.

12. Pedersen TR, Kjekhus J, Berg K, et al. Cholesterol lowering and the use of healthcare resources. Results of the Scandinavian Simvastatin Survival Study. *Circulation* 1996; **93**: 1796–802.

13. Mihaylova B, Briggs A, Armitage J, et al. Cost-effectiveness of simvastatin in people at different levels of vascular disease risk: economic analysis of a randomised trial in 20,536 individuals. *Lancet* 2005; **365**: 1779–85.

14. Shepherd J, Blauw GJ, Murphy MB, et al. Pravastatin in elderly individuals at risk of vascular disease (PROSPER): a randomised controlled trial. *Lancet* 2002; **360**: 1623–30.

15. Heart Protection Study Collaborative Group. MRC/BHF heart protection study of cholesterol lowering with simvastatin in 20536 high-risk individuals: a randomised placebo-controlled trial. *Lancet* 2002; **360**: 7–22.

16. Myant NB. *The Biology of Cholesterol and Related Sterols.* London: Heinemann, 1981.

17. Consumer Reports. The statin drugs, 2006. Available at: www.CRBestBuyDrugs.org.

18. DiMasi JA, Hansen RW, Grabowski HG. The price of innovation: new estimates of drug development costs. *J Health Econ* 2003; **22**: 151–85.

19. Francis Bacon. *The Advancement of Learning.* First published in 1605; revised edition: New York: Modern Library, 2001.

Glossary of abbreviations, acronyms and scientific terms

ABC ATP-binding cassette
ADG Atherosclerosis Discussion Group
adrenergic mediated by adrenaline
aetiology the cause of a disease
albumin the major protein in plasma
aldosterone the hormone regulating sodium and potassium metabolism
α-lipoprotein original term for high-density lipoprotein
anacetrapib a CETP inhibitor
angina chest pain due to insufficient blood flow to myocardium (heart muscle)
angiographic radiographic visualization of arteries with a contrast medium
anti-hypertensive blood pressure-lowering medication
anti-platelet inhibitor of platelet activity
aortic valve valve located at base of the aorta
apolipoprotein protein component of a lipoprotein
arterial intima inner lining of artery
atheroma cholesterol-rich core of an atherosclerotic plaque
atherosclerosis the pathological process underlying coronary heart disease
atherosclerotic plaque lipid and/or fibrous lesion within the intima of large and medium-sized arteries
atorvastatin a synthetic HMG CoA reductase inhibitor
ATP adenosine triphosphate
Atromid proprietary name for clofibrate
AUC area under the curve
azole a nitrogen-containing chemical compound

β-carotene a fat-soluble provitamin
β-lipoprotein original term for low-density lipoprotein
BAS British Atherosclerosis Society
BHF British Heart Foundation
bile acid sequestrant anion-exchange resin that binds bile salts
biopsy tissue sample

bleeding time measure of platelet activity

^{14}C a radioactive isotope of carbon
campestanol a plant stanol
campesterol a plant sterol
carcinogenic cancer inducing
carotid main artery to the head and brain
catabolic degradative
cerivastatin a synthetic HMG CoA reductase inhibitor
CETP cholesterol ester transfer protein
chlorphenoxyisobutyric acid pharmacologically active
    constituent of clofibrate
cholesterol the major sterol found in mammals
cholestyramine a bile acid sequestrant used to lower cholesterol
chylomicron a large lipoprotein which transports absorbed fat from
    the small intestine into the bloodstream
CK creatine phosphokinase (an enzyme released by damaged muscle)
clofibrate generic name for chlorphenoxyisobutyric acid
coeliac disease intestinal malabsorption syndrome resulting from
    gluten intolerance
colestipol a bile acid sequestrant used to lower cholesterol
collagen protein constituent of fibrous tissue
COMA Committee on the Medical Aspects [of Food Policy]
compactin the first HMG CoA reductase inhibitor
continuous flow blood cell separator centrifugal device for
    extracorporeal separation of blood cells from plasma
coronary heart disease clinical consequences of coronary
    atherosclerosis
cortisol hormone synthesized by the adrenal cortex
CPPT Coronary Primary Prevention Trial
creatine phosphokinase *see CK*
cyclosporine immunosuppressive drug
CYP3A4 cytochrome P450 3A4
CYP2C8 cytochrome P450 2C8
cytochrome P450 liver enzyme complex involved in drug
    metabolism

DNA deoxyribonucleic acid
double bond chemical bond in which two pairs of electrons link
    two atoms
dyslipoproteinaemia abnormal state of plasma lipoproteins

ECG electrocardiogram
electrolytes ionized constituents of plasma
electrophoresis method of separating proteins with an electric
    current
ENHANCE trial examining the effect of combination ezetimibe and
    high-dose simvastatin vs simvastatin alone on the atherosclerotic
    process
EPIC European Prospective Investigation of Cancer

epidemiology study of the incidence and distribution of diseases
essential fatty acid unsaturated fatty acid which cannot be
  synthesized and so must be obtained from food to maintain
  health
esterified linkage of an acid with an alkyl or other organic group,
  such as oleic acid with cholesterol
esters end result of the esterification process
ezetimibe a cholesterol absorption inhibitor

FATS Familial Atherosclerosis Treatment Study
fatty acid hydrocarbon with a variable number of carbon atoms
  and a terminal carboxyl group
fatty streak earliest stage of the atherosclerotic process
FDA (US) Food and Drug Administration
fenofibrate a fibric acid derivative
FH familial hypercholesterolaemia
fibrinogen plasma protein essential for blood clotting
fibroblast connective tissue cell which produces collagen
fluvastatin a synthetic HMG CoA reductase inhibitor
Folch extraction method of extracting lipids from tissue or plasma
4S Scandinavian Simvastatin Survival Study

gemfibrozil a fibric acid derivative
genarylgenarylation a type of lipid modification (prenylation)
  involving covalent addition of isoprenoids to proteins
glucose tolerance ability to maintain normal blood glucose levels
glucuronidation metabolic process whereby the liver or intestine
  combines drugs with glucuronic acid prior to excretion
GRAS generally regarded as safe

haemodynamic pertaining to blood flow
HDL high-density lipoprotein
heterozygote person inheriting one normal and one mutant allele
  of a specific gene
HMG CoA hydroxymethylglutaryl co-enzyme A
HMG CoA reductase the rate-limiting enzyme of cholesterol
  synthesis
homozygous inheritance of two mutant alleles of a specific gene
HPS Heart Protection Study
hydrogenated combined with hydrogen (hydrogenation is a
  catalytic process whereby liquid fats are solidified)
hydrolysis chemical breakdown by reaction with water
hypercholesterolaemia high concentration of cholesterol in the
  blood
hyperlipidaemia high concentration of lipids in the blood
hyperlipoproteinaemia high concentration of lipoproteins in the
  blood
hypertension high blood pressure

^{125}**I** a radioactive isotope of iodine emitting β-particles

^{131}I a gamma ray-emitting isotope of iodine
ICI Imperial Chemical Industries
ILLUMINATE Investigation of Lipid Level Management to Understand its Impact in Atherosclerotic Events [trial]
ILLUSTRATE Investigation of Lipid Level Management Using Coronary Ultrasound to Assess Reduction of Atherosclerosis by CETP inhibition and HDL Elevation [trial]
IMPROVE-IT Improved Reduction of Outcomes: VYTORIN Efficacy International Trial
IMT intima-medial thickness
infarct area of dead tissue resulting from an interrupted blood supply
insulin hormone involved in glucose homeostasis
ischaemic inadequate blood supply
ischaemic heart disease synonymous with coronary heart disease

jugular venous pressure level of filling of external jugular vein, used as an indicator of heart failure

LASA Longitudinal Aging Study Amsterdam
LDL low-density lipoprotein
LDL receptor the main determinant of plasma cholesterol concentration
linoleic acid an essential polyunsaturated fatty acid
lipid fatty substance such as cholesterol, triglyceride or free fatty acid
lipidology speciality dealing with disorders of lipid metabolism
lipopolysaccharide large molecule consisting of lipid covalently linked to carbohydrate
lipoproteins varying types of water-miscible particles formed by interaction of apolipoproteins with lipids
liquid scintillation counting method of estimating the amount of radioactivity in samples
lovastatin an HMG CoA reductase inhibitor produced by fermentation
LRC Lipid Research Clinics
lumen central cavity of hollow tube

macrolide antibiotics containing multiple lactone rings
macrophage type of inflammatory cell
meta-analysis statistical analysis of pooled data from a number of trials
metabolism biochemical processes which maintain life
mevastatin alternative name for compactin
mevinolin original name for lovastatin
MGH Massachusetts General Hospital
mixed micelles complexes of bile salts, fatty acids and monoglycerides
MONICA Monitoring Trends and Determinants in Cardiovascular Disease

monocolin K an HMG CoA reductase inhibitor identical to lovastatin
MRC Medical Research Council
mucosa membranous lining
myocardial infarct ischaemic damage to heart muscle (heart attack)
myositis inflamed or damaged muscle
myotoxic causing myositis

neuronal of nerve cell origin
NHS National Health Service
NICE National Institute for Health and Clinical Excellence
nicotinic acid B group vitamin used in high doses to treat dyslipidaemia
NIH (US) National Institutes of Health

oleic acid non-essential monounsaturated fatty acid
ω-3 fatty acid long-chain polyunsaturated fatty acids of marine or plant origin with three or more double bonds

partial ileal bypass surgical diversion of intestinal contents past distal small intestine to prevent bile acid reabsorption and lower blood cholesterol
pectin polysaccharide present in ripe fruit
pectinase enzyme which breaks down pectin
pharmacokinetics the absorption, distribution and excretion of drugs
phenotypic outward expression of genotype interacting with environment
phospholipid major constituent of cell membranes and lipoproteins
phytosterol general term encompassing plant sterols and stanols
placebo inert comparator used in drug trials
plant stanols saturated plant sterols
plant sterols cholesterol-like compounds of vegetable origin
plasma the liquid component of blood
plasma exchange therapeutic exchange of plasma for albumin solution
plasmapheresis literally means 'taking away plasma' and is used synonymously with plasma exchange
platelets blood cells that arrest bleeding and promote coagulation
pleiotropic multiple, unrelated effects
polyunsaturated fatty acid possessing two or more double bonds
pravastatin an HMG CoA reductase inhibitor derived from microbial fermentation
preparative ultracentrifugation process used to separate lipoproteins of differing density
primary prevention prevention of disease before it is clinically apparent
PROCAM Prospective Cardiovascular Munster [Study]

progression enlargement of atherosclerotic plaques
PROSPER Prospective Study of Pravastatin in the Elderly at Risk
pulmonary embolus blockage of a branch of the pulmonary artery
by a clot dislodged from a peripheral vein

QALY quality-adjusted life year
QCA quantitative coronary angiography

RADIANCE 1 Rating Atherosclerotic Disease Change by Imaging
with a New CETP Inhibitor [trial]
regression trials angiographic trials designed to assess effect of
lipid-lowering therapy on coronary atherosclerosis
revascularization enhancing coronary blood supply by surgically
bypassing or by dilating atheromatous lesions
rhabdomyolysis massive breakdown of muscle leading to
myoglobinuria
rosuvastatin a synthetic HMG CoA reductase inhibitor

saturated fat consists of fatty acids lacking double bonds
secondary prevention preventing the worsening or recurrence of
disease in subjects already manifesting the disorder
serotoninergic mediated by the neurotransmitter serotonin
side chain chain of carbon atoms linked to steroid nucleus of sterols
simvastatin an HMG CoA reductase inhibitor derived by microbial
fermentation
sitostanol a plant stanol
sitosterol a plant sterol
sitosterolaemia a rare inherited disorder characterized by excessive
absorption of plant sterols
squalene synthase an enzyme acting further down the cholesterol
synthetic pathway than HMG CoA reductase
statin synonymous with HMG CoA reductase inhibitor
stenosed narrowed
stenosis narrowing
sterol unsaturated steroid alcohol
systolic phase of the cardiac cycle when the ventricles contract

tendon xanthoma thickening of tendon due to sterol
accumulation
thin-layer chromatography method of separating lipids using
silica plates
thrombosis formation of a blood clot
thyroid endocrine gland in the neck
thyroxine hormone from thyroid gland which regulates metabolic
rate
torcetrapib a CETP inhibitor
trans-fatty acids hardened fats formed by partial hydrogenation of
mono- or polyunsaturated fatty acids
triglyceride a major plasma lipid and the chief constituent of
adipose tissue

tropical sprue a form of fat malabsorption occurring in the tropics
t-**test** a test of statistical significance

ubiquinone a product of HMG CoA reductase, also known as co-enzyme Q10
uric acid end product of purine metabolism, excess of which causes gout

VA-HIT Veterans Affairs HDL cholesterol Intervention Trial
vitamin D fat-soluble vitamin essential for bone calcification
VLDL very low-density lipoprotein

WHO World Health Organization
WOSCOPS West of Scotland Coronary Prevention Study

Index